ABC OF COLORECTAL DISEASES
SECOND EDITION

ABC OF COLORECTAL DISEASES

SECOND EDITION

edited by

D J JONES

Consultant General and Colorectal Surgeon, Wythenshawe Hospital,
South Manchester University Hospitals NHS Trust

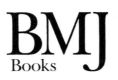

The cover image shows cancer of the colon, and is reproduced with permission from the Science Photo Library. Coloured barium enema x-ray of the human abdomen showing a cancer of the asending colon; the tumour appears as the oval shadow over the right pelvic bone (left on image). Opaque to x-rays, barium is given orally (barium meal) for investigations of the oesophagus, stomach and duodenum and rectally (as barium enema) to examine the rectum and colon. The colon (large intestine) consists of four sections–the ascending, transverse, descending and sigmoid colons. Here, the ascending colon rises left, its traverse (horizontal) section appears centre and with the descending part at right, which connects with the rectum via the sigmoid colon.

© BMJ Books, 1999
BMJ Books is an imprint of the BMJ Publishing Group

First edition published in 1993
by the BMJ Publishing Group, BMA House,
Tavistock Square, London WC1H 9JR
Second edition 1999

British Library Cataloguing in Publication Data

A catalogue record for this book is avaialble from the British Library

ISBN 0-7279-1105-8

Typeset by Apek Typesetters, Nailsea, Bristol
Printed and bound by Clifford Press

Contents

CONTRIBUTORS

G L Carlson
Senior Lecturer in Surgery, Hope Hospital, Salford

N M Craven
Clinical Lecturer and Honorary Senior Registrar, Hope Hospital, Salford

C M Doig
Senior Lecturer in Paediatric Surgery, University of Manchester, Booth Hall, Children's Hospital, Manchester

B P Goorney
Consultant Physician, Department of Genitourinary Medicine, Hope Hospital, Salford

B D Hancock
Consultant General and Colorectal Surgeon, Wythenshawe Hospital, Manchester

J Hill
Consultant General and Colorectal Surgeon, Manchester Royal Infirmary, Manchester

J H Hobbiss
Consultant General and Colorectal Surgeon, Bolton General Hospital

S Hughes
Colorectal Nurse Specialist, Hope Hospital, Salford

M H Irving
Professor of Surgery, Hope Hospital, Salford

R D James
Consultant Radiotherapist, Christie Hospital and Holt Radium Institute, Manchester

D J Jones
Consultant General and Colorectal Surgeon, Wythenshawe Hospital, Manchester

E S Kiff
Consultant General and Colorectal Surgeon, Wythenshawe Hospital, Manchester

B K Mandal
Consultant Physician, Department of Infectious Diseases and Tropical Medicine, Monsall Unit, North Manchester General Hospital

K J Moriarty
Consultant Gastroenterologist, Bolton General Hospital

N O'Donoghue
Senior House Officer in Gastroenterology, General Bolton Hospital

S T O'Dwyer
Consultant Colorectal Surgeon, Christie Hospital and Holt Radium Institute, Manchester

P F Schofield
Professor of Surgery, Manchester

N A Scott
Consultant General and Colorectal Surgeon, Hope Hosptial, Salford

J L Shaffer
Consultant Gastroenterologist, Hope Hospital, Salford

D G Thompson
Professor of Gastroenterology, Hope Hospital, Salford

A J M Watson
Professor of Medicine, Royal Liverpool Hospital, Liverpool

INTRODUCTION

This book brings together the articles that were published in the *BMJ*. The authors are surgeons and physicians, mainly from the Manchester School, with an active clinical and research interest in their particular subject. We have revised and updated the chapters, taking into account the helpful comments and interest we received following their initial publication.

Colorectal diseases are common, and patients may present to doctors in almost any sphere of medical practice. Minor anorectal problems such as haemorrhoids may be regarded by doctor and patient as being of little consequence, but they can cause considerable distress and may indicate serious underlying pathology. Most anorectal conditions fortunately are easily diagnosed and can be effectively treated.

We have written the book primarily for general practitioners and clinicians without a specialist training in coloproctology and for gastrointestinal physicians and surgeons in training. The aim has been to provide the essential knowledge to make a diagnosis, initiate appropriate treatment or referral, and to provide the background information necessary to understand the patient's further management. We hope the book will also be of value to medical students and nursing colleagues in the United Kingdom and overseas.

D J JONES
Wythenshawe Hospital
Manchester

ACKNOWLEDGMENTS

The line drawings throughout the book were prepared by Paul Somerset, Department of Medical Illustration, Wythenshawe Hospital, Manchester. The photographs were prepared by the Department of Medical Illustration, Salford Royal Hospitals NHS Trust and the Department of Medical Illustration, Wythenshawe Hospital, South Manchester University Hospitals NHS Trust, unless otherwise stated.

1   Anatomy and physiology of the colon, rectum, and anus

J Hill, M H Irving

Anatomy

The large bowel is 1·5 m long, with an antireflux ileocaecal valve at its proximal end and the dentate line of the anal canal at its distal end. The transverse colon always has a mesentery, the ascending colon has a mesentery in only 12% of people, and the descending colon has one in 22%. The sigmoid colon also has a mesentery and is sometimes unusually long (dolicolon)—a feature that predisposes to volvulus. The luminal surface of the colon is lined with mucosa rich in mucus secreting goblet cells. Deep into the mucosa are the muscularis mucosa, submucosa, and the outer muscular coat—the muscularis propria. This muscle layer has an inner continuous circular layer and an outer longitudinal muscle layer which is condensed into three bands—the taenia coli.

Blood supply to the colon

The superior mesenteric artery supplies blood to the right colon as far as the distal transverse colon. The left colon and upper rectum are supplied by the inferior mesenteric artery, and the remainder of the rectum and anal canal by the middle rectal arteries and branches of the pudendal arteries. Arterial disease of the aorta may often narrow or even occlude the mesenteric arteries, particularly the inferior mesenteric artery, in which event the circulation is maintained by the superior mesenteric artery via the anastomosis near the gut wall—the so called marginal artery. Of the smaller arteries, those of the transverse colon seem especially liable to atherosclerosis.

The venous drainage from the right colon is predominantly to the right hepatic lobe and from the rectum and left colon to the left hepatic lobe owing to the "streaming" of blood in the portal vein. The lymphatic vessels pass into small glands located along the colonic wall, then on to intermediate lymph nodes on the main colic vessels, and their branches; then they pass on to the principal glands along the superior and inferior mesenteric artery and aorta.

Nerve supply to the colon

The smooth muscle fibres of the colonic wall are in direct communication with each other through gap junctions; their activity is further coordinated by an intramural nerve plexus and connections from the extrinsic nerves. Sympathetic nerves pass from the aortic plexus along the arteries. These nerves carry inhibitory impulses to the muscular coats of the colon and rectum, and vasoconstrictor fibres. There are possibly also some stimulatory fibres. Bilateral extensive sympathectomy abolishes visceral pain.

The main motor or parasympathetic fibres come from the vagus nerve to the part of the gut supplied by the superior mesenteric artery. More distally the gut receives parasympathetic nerves from the sacral outflow, which run with the inferior mesenteric vessels and supply the bowel wall as far as the distal transverse colon.

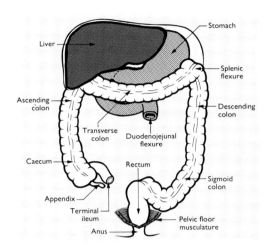

Figure 1.1   The large bowel

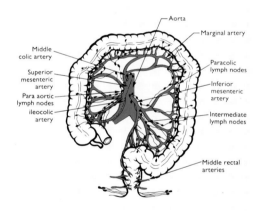

Figure 1.2   Blood supply and lymphatic drainage

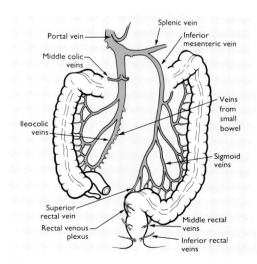

Figure 1.3   Venous drainage

1

Functions of the colon

The principal functions of the colon are to remove water from the one litre of ileal effluent that enters it each day, and to store faeces. Water, electrolytes, and some metabolites are removed by the mucous membrane which is moved over the luminal content by local and total wall contraction. Potassium is added to the content by mucus secretion. Ingested cellulose is excreted unchanged; a high fibre diet helps to retain water and increase the faecal bulk, thus aiding defecation.

The intrinsic nerve plexus is required for colorectal contraction as shown by its partial absence in the congenital Hirschsprung's disease, its destruction by trypanosomes in Chagas' disease, and prolonged drug taking—for example, of chlorpromazine or senna—all leading to obstruction or severe constipation.

The intrinsic plexus is, however, under the influence of gut and other hormones the varying circulating concentrations of which significantly affect the contractile activity. For example, cholecystokinin, motilin, and gastrin all stimulate motor activity, whereas vasoactive intestinal peptide, glucagon, and secretin are inhibitory. Thus, after meals motility rises considerably under the influence of the extrinsic nervous plexus and also perhaps because of cholecystokinin activity. Sleep greatly reduces colonic activity which increases immediately on awakening. Mental stress also increases colonic activity.

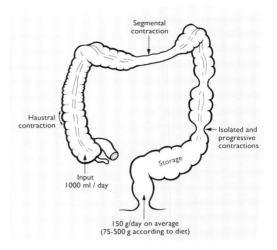

Figure 1.5   Activity of large bowel

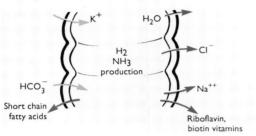

Figure 1.4   Absorption (blue arrows) and secretion (red arrows) in the large bowel

Drugs

Many drugs have a potent effect on colonic motility, by either stimulation or inhibition of receptors on the smooth muscle itself or on neural tissue supplying smooth muscle, or by interfering with the influx of calcium into cells (calcium channel blockers). Thus normal bowel tone may be increased or depressed to produce diarrhoea or functional obstruction. Both reduction of serum potassium concentrations and inhibition by slow calcium channel blockers can have a profound effect on smooth muscle function.

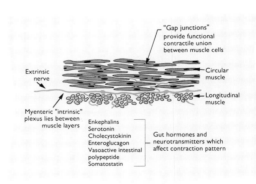

Figure 1.6   Intramural autonomic nerve plexus

Rectum and anus

The rectum turns downwards and backwards from the rectosigmoid junction to follow the curve of the sacrum. It passes out of the peritoneal cavity to end 2 cm in front of and below the tip of the coccyx at its junction with the anal canal. The rectum is totally sheathed in longitudinal muscle fibres. The colorectum is lined with columnar epithelium as far as the dentate line in the middle of the anal canal, where sensitive squamous epithelium, in continuity with that of the perineal skin, takes over. In normal subjects there is a 60–105° angle between the rectum and anal canal. This angle is maintained by the puborectalis muscle which passes backwards from the pubis around the anorectal junction and back to the pubis, so pulling the anorectal junction forwards.

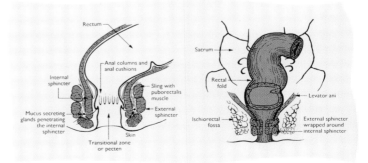

Figure 1.7   Anteroposterior (left) and lateral view (right) of rectum and anus

The anal canal is slightly shorter in women than in men (mean 3·7 cm vs 4·6 cm). It is surrounded by two cylinders of muscle, the internal anal sphincter (comprised of smooth muscle fibres) responsible for 80% of the resting tone, and the external anal sphincter. The external sphincter works in harmony with the puborectalis and levator ani of the pelvic floor. This voluntary sphincter complex can double the resting tone in the anal canal (squeeze pressure). Normally the internal sphincter seems to have a cyclic (15/minute) pattern of contraction. As the frequency of contraction is higher distally in the canal, this may assist continence and anal cleanliness by retrograde propulsion. The soft vascular submucosal tissue above the dentate line, which on hypertrophy produces haemorrhoids, also aids occlusion of the canal. Submucous anal glands may extend deeply into the sphincter and, if infected, may lead to perianal abscess and fistula.

Defecation

The rectum is normally empty; wakening and ingestion of food lead to an increase in left colon motility, and faeces entering the rectum result in a call to stool. Sitting on the toilet helps to straighten out the anorectal angle, a process aided by relaxation of the voluntary sphincter complex, and faeces enter the anal canal, to be passed if the passage is not voluntarily stopped. During defecation the internal anal sphincter relaxes as part of the rectoanal inhibitory reflex. Anorectal sensation permits discrimination of solid from gas. Further faeces from as far cephalad as the splenic flexure may be passed. The average daily volume is 150 ml.

The rectum can accommodate passively a volume of 400 ml, maintaining a low rectal pressure. Chronic tolerance of faeces in the rectum may be associated with severe constipation.

Maintenance of continence is dependent on several major factors:

- An effective barrier to outflow provided by anal sphincters and perhaps an acute anorectal angle
- A capacious, passively distensible, and evacuable reservoir
- Intact rectal and anal sensation
- Intact central neurological function
- Bulky and formed faeces.

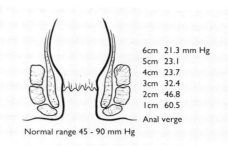
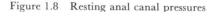

6cm	21.3 mm Hg
5cm	23.1
4cm	23.7
3cm	32.4
2cm	46.8
1cm	60.5
	Anal verge

Normal range 45 - 90 mm Hg

Figure 1.8   Resting anal canal pressures

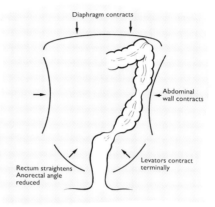

Figure 1.9   Mechanism of defacation

- Faeces enter rectum
- Reflex relaxation of sphincter
- Intra-abdominal pressure rises
- Anorectal angle straightens
- Gut contraction empties left colon into rectum
- Faeces squeezed through anus

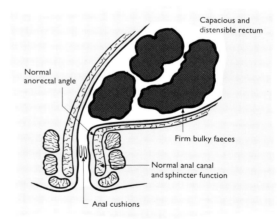

Figure 1.10   Factors necessary for anal continence

2 Investigation of colorectal disorders

D J Jones, M H Irving

When investigating a patient for colorectal disorders a detailed history is important and will provide clues to the diagnosis. Symptoms arising from the large bowel tend to be non-specific and are often difficult to interpret. There is a wide variation in bowel habit, so alterations from a patient's normal bowel pattern, changes in longstanding symptoms, and the passage of blood and mucus are of most importance.

Colorectal disorders are associated with several systemic manifestations which may hint at the underlying diagnosis: anaemia is associated with neoplasia and inflammatory bowel disease; dermoid cysts with Gardner's syndrome; acanthosis nigricans and dermatomyositis with neoplasia; and pyoderma gangrenosum, arthropathy, uveitis, and finger clubbing all with inflammatory bowel disease.

Symptoms of colorectal disorders

General—Malaise; weight loss; vomiting

Abdominal—pain (constant or colic); distension; borborygmi

Bowel habit—Altered frequency; constipation; diarrhoea; taking laxative and antidiarrhoeal drugs; stool consistency; bleeding (bright red, mixed in motion, dark, altered); slime (mucus)

Anal and perineal—Pruritus; pain and its relation to defecation; prolapse; incontinence; discharge; tenesmus; swelling (painful or painless)

Abdominal examination

Ideally the patient should be comfortable, relaxed, and supine for abdominal examination. The abdomen should be inspected for distension and visible peristalsis. Gentle palpation will often reveal a palpable sigmoid colon, which can be considered a normal finding in constipated patients. Diverticular disease and colonic cancer may manifest as palpable masses. Palpation of the liver may disclose secondary spread in patients with colorectal cancer.

The characteristic rebound tenderness associated with peritonitis should be elicited by gentle percussion and not by the sudden release of a deeply palpating hand, which is less sensitive and causes extreme discomfort in patients with peritonitis.

Differential diagnosis of lower abdominal mass

Left iliac fossa
- Carcinonoma of the sigmoid colon
- Diverticular disease

Right iliac fossa
- Carcinoma of the caecum
- Crohn's disease
- Abscess of the appendix
- Ileocaecal tuberculosis
- Actinomycosis
- Intussusception

Either iliac fossa
- Ovarian mass
- Ectopic kidney
- Transplanted kidney

Anorectal examination

The rectum and anus are readily accessible, so their clinical examination is often the mainstay of diagnosis. Few patients relish this examination, which should be indicated and not performed "routinely". Patients feel embarrassed and exposed, and anxiety provokes spasm of the anal sphincters and buttocks. This is exacerbated by a rough technique, which results in an unpleasant examination with little yield. Fears are allayed by prior explanation. Patients should be placed in the left lateral position with a pillow under the hip and covered with a blanket. They are warned that although they may feel they are losing control of their continence during the examination, an "accident" is unlikely.

Digital examination

Examination begins with inspection of the anus under good lighting. Many pathological conditions such as skin tags in Crohn's disease are immediately obvious and may indicate underlying rectal or colonic pathology. The state of anal tone is observed at rest and on voluntary contraction. The patient is asked to "strain down", as if defecating, to show perineal descent, prolapsing haemorrhoids, or protruding lesions such as rectal prolapse and tumours.

Findings on anal inspection
- Pruritus ani
- Perianal warts
- Perianal abscess
- Perianal haematoma
- Prolapsing haemorrhoids
- Thrombosed haemorrhoids
- Skin tags
- Anal fistulas
- Anal fissures
- Anal cancer
- Rectocele
- Rectal prolapse
- Faecal soiling of perineum

A gloved lubricated finger is placed flat on the anus. Gentle pressure is applied until the sphincter yields and the finger glides into the anus. The rectal contents and mucosa within reach of the finger are palpated. The prostate or cervix is noted, together with any extrarectal lesions. The patient is asked to tighten the anus to assess sphincter tone, and the puborectal muscle is felt by hooking the finger over it. If lesions are discovered their mobility over the surrounding tissues is assessed. Chronic anal fissures and induration from fistulas may be felt, but haemorrhoids are not usually palpable. The withdrawn finger is inspected for blood, mucus, and pus, and the nature of the faeces noted.

Proctoscopy

After digital examination the anal canal is inspected with a proctoscope. A disposable proctoscope with fibreoptic lighting is preferred. It is inserted with the obturator in place, until the sphincter resistance is overcome, after which the obturator is removed. The lower rectal mucosa is seen and the proctoscope slowly withdrawn, showing the haemorrhoidal cushions, the dentate line, and the anal epithelium. It is useful to ask the patient to "bear down" during withdrawal in order to demonstrate prolapsing mucosa and haemorrhoids. The examination may need to be repeated for complete assessment.

Sigmoidoscopy

Rigid sigmoidoscopy—This is easily performed in the outpatient clinic, and only in exceptional circumstances is a general anaesthetic necessary. The initial examination should be without bowel preparation, which is irritant and may evoke changes mimicking proctitis. Complete visualisation of the rectum is usually possible, but a disposable phosphate enema may help if the rectum is loaded with faeces. The instrument is introduced in the same manner as the proctoscope and slowly advanced along the lumen of the rectum, displacing the mucosal folds by gentle inflation and angulation of the instrument. The tip of the sigmoidoscope should be advanced only when the lumen ahead is visible. It is usually possible to negotiate the rectosigmoid angulation, but care is needed to reduce discomfort and pain from distortion of the anus and stretching of the colonic wall. Biopsy samples of protuberant lesions can be taken with impunity, but mucosal lesions should be biopsied only below 10 cm with rigid biopsy instruments. Rupture of the rectum during sigmoidoscopy is inexcusable.

Flexible sigmoidoscopy—Flexible fibreoptic sigmoidoscopy allows examination up to 60 cm from the anal margin and can usually be performed without sedation in less than 10 minutes. Bowel preparation with a disposable phosphate enema is usually sufficient. Fibreoptic instruments are more expensive than rigid sigmoidoscopes and need more complex cleansing and maintenance by specially trained staff, and they are less suited to a busy outpatient clinic. The yield of pathological abnormalities is, however, greater than with rigid instruments and about 70% of colorectal carcinomas are within reach of the flexible sigmoidoscope.

Colonoscopy

Colonoscopy is a skilled procedure which requires specialist training. Bowel preparation is essential and several regimens have been described. Patients should take a low residue diet followed by clear fluids for 48 hours before colonoscopy, and take a strong purgative such as sodium picosulphate on the morning and evening of the day before colonoscopy. Mannitol produces rapid bowel preparation, but produces hydrogen, which is potentially explosive if electrocautery or snaring is

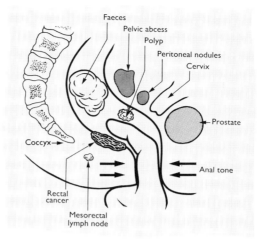

Figure 2.1   Findings on rectal examination.

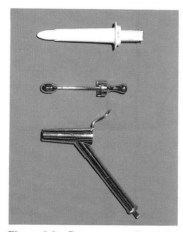

Figure 2.2   Proctoscopes: Top: disposable proctoscope; middle: obturator for proctoscope; bottom: reusable metal proctoscope.

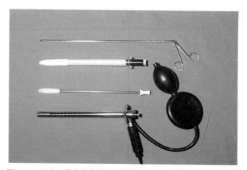

Figure 2.3   Rigid sigmoidoscopes (from top to bottom): biopsy forceps; disposable sigmoidoscope; obturator for sigmoidoscope; metal reusable sigmoidoscope with connected light source and bellows for insuflation.

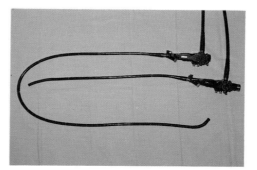

Figure 2.4 Outer: colonoscope; central: flexible sigmoidoscope.

used. Caution is needed in patients with possible obstruction, for whom large volume enemas are more appropriate than strong purgatives. Colonoscopy is usually performed under light sedation with either midazolam or diazepam. This is often supplemented with an antispasmodic drug (for example, hyoscine butylbromide) and an analgesic such as pethidine. The technique induces hypoxia, so the patient's oxygen saturation should be monitored by pulse oximetry and oxygen given as required. Experienced colonoscopists reach the caecum in 90% or more of cases.

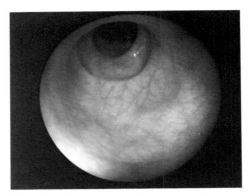

Figure 2.5 Normal colon viewed through a colonoscope.

Barium enema examination

A single contrast barium enema examination is inaccurate and shows only extreme abnormalities. A limited examination may be used to confirm mechanical blockage and exclude pseudo-obstruction before operating for suspected large bowel obstruction. A double contrast barium enema examination entails insufflation of air after evacuation of barium. This provides fine mucosal detail and the diagnostic accuracy approaches that of colonoscopy. Double contrast barium enema examination will disclose gross anatomy and extra-colonic abnormalities such as fistulas that are not easily seen on endoscopy. Colonoscopy is more sensitive for detecting fine mucosal abnormalities; biopsy samples can be taken and therapeutic procedures such as polypectomy performed. The choice of investigation may be dictated by the availability of local resources and expertise.

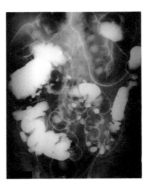

Figure 2.6 Double contrast barium enema showing diverticular disease.

Imaging

Preoperative abdominal ultrasonography may show clinically inapparent metastases in patients with colorectal cancer.

Preoperative computed tomography and magnetic resonance scanning provide more accurate information about the local extent of rectal cancers and are more sensitive at detecting hepatic metastases than abdominal ultrasonography. Intraoperative ultrasonography is, however, emerging as the most sensitive imaging technique for detecting hepatic metastases.

Magnetic resonance imaging is particularly useful in the assessment of complex anal fistulas. Endoanal ultrasonography (EUS) is emerging as a useful way of demonstrating anal sphincter defects. It may also have a role in assessing the depths of spread in low rectal and anal cancers and help select patients suitable for local resection and radiotherapy.

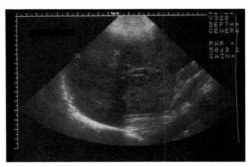

Figure 2.7 Ultrasound scan showing hepatic metastases.

Faeces

The detection of occult blood in the faeces is important in the investigation of patients with unexplained iron deficiency anaemia and forms the basis of screening for colorectal cancer. Haemoccult is the most widely used test for screening. The patient smears faeces on a filter impregnated with guaiac acid. This is returned to the laboratory, where hydrogen peroxide is added. If haematin from haemoglobin is present in the faeces it catalyses the oxidation of guaiac acid, giving a characteristic colour change to blue. Immunological tests with antibodies specific for human haemoglobin may prove to be more sensitive.

If infection is suspected fresh samples of faeces should be obtained for microbiological examination. Microscopy will show any mobile amoebas and parasitic cysts; culture will grow bacterial pathogens. Toxins produced by *Clostridium difficile* may be identified in patients with pseudomembranous colitis.

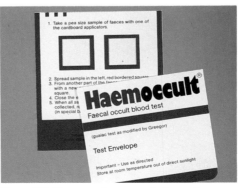

Figure 2.8 Haemoccult test card; the patient smears faeces on the test squares. Hydrogen peroxide is applied in the laboratory. A blue colour change indicates occult blood in the faeces.

Anorectal function tests

The objective assessment of anorectal physiology is playing an expanding part in the understanding and management of patients with faecal incontinence, sphincter injuries, rectal prolapse, and abnormalities of defecation. The pathogenesis of these disorders is incompletely understood and the full significance of many of these measurements uncertain at present.

Anal manometry is performed, preferably by using air filled or, more commonly, water perfused balloon systems. Solid state transducers are more convenient but less reliable. Maximum resting and squeeze pressures are recorded, which measure internal and external sphincter mechanism function, respectively. Pressures decrease with age and they are commonly reduced in incontinent patients. Rectal compliance is measured by filling a rectal baloon and recording the volume and pressure at first sensation and noting the maximum capacity the patient will tolerate. Patients with inflammatory conditions have decreased compliance, while those with faecal impaction and constipation may tolerate large volumes and high pressures. Sphincter motor nerve function and muscle activity are assessed by electromyography with fine electrodes. This information is of help in mapping sphincter defects which may be repairable. Neuropathic damage to the pudendal nerve is assessed by measuring pundendal nerve motor latency, which is the time taken for an impulse to travel from the ischial spine to the sphincter.

The rectoanal reflex causes a reduction in resting pressure when filling a rectal balloon, representing reflex inhibition of sphincter contraction. The reflex is lost in patients with Hirschsprung's disease owing to aganglionosis and may be absent in patients with rectal prolapse and incontinence if resting pressures are already low.

Anal sensation is measured by applying an electric current or thermal stimulus to the anal epithelium until the threshold of sensation is reached. Loss of sensation may be important in the aetiology of incontinence in patients who have had previous anorectal surgery.

Proctography with barium suspensions is used to measure the anorectal angle. Patients with incontinence often have obtuse angles secondary to pelvic floor weakness. A videoproctogram records the expulsion of a thick barium suspension, simulating defecation, and will show prolapse, rectoceles, and the function of ileoanal reservoirs. Colonic transit is studied by ingestion of special radio-opaque markers, which can be followed by plain abdominal radiography.

Endoanal ultrasonography is a useful adjunct to these investigations because it demonstrates defects in the anal sphincters.

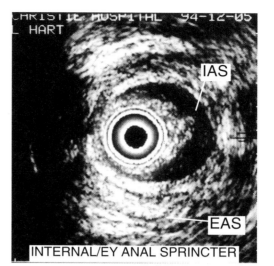

Figure 2.9 Endoanal ultrasound scan.
(IAS) Internal anal sphincter
(EAS) External anal sphincter

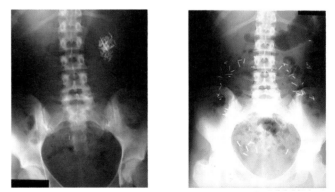

Figure 2.10 Plain abdominal radiographs showing the progress of ingested radio-opaque markers used to evaluate colonic transit time, which is prolonged in slow transit constipation.

3 Constipation

K J Moriarty, N O'Donoghue

There is considerable geographical and racial variation in bowel habit. Constipation is largely a subjective sensation and it has no universally accepted definition. A reasonable working definition is straining at passing stools for more than 25% of bowel movements.

Figure 3.1 shows the relationship between fibre intake in three populations, transit time, and stool weight.

Mechanisms of defecation

The function of the colon is to mix and propel its contents and to absorb water and electrolytes. Colonic and rectal motilities are regulated by the sympathetic, parasympathetic, and enteric nervous systems, and thus lesions of those pathways will influence stool frequency. Colonic motility is stimulated by factors such as food and emotion. The presence of sufficient faeces in the rectum to cause distension leads to reflex contraction of rectal smooth muscle and relaxation of the internal anal sphincter. By contracting the diaphragm and abdominal muscles, and relaxing the striated muscles of the puborectalis and external anal sphincter, the stool can be expelled.

Assessment of constipation

The assessment of constipation is based on a consideration of the possible causes. Simple constipation is infrequent or irregular defecation which may be painful and is not secondary to an underlying cause. It typically occurs in young women who commonly have a low intake of dietary fibre. It may also occur in those who ignore the need to pass stools, in shift workers, and because of lack of exercise. Anorectal disorders are diagnosed by inspection and digital examination of the rectum, together with proctoscopy and sigmoidoscopy.

Diverticular disease and colonic tumours are diagnosed by double contrast barium enema examination or colonoscopy. These disorders should be considered, particularly in older patients presenting with a change in bowel habit.

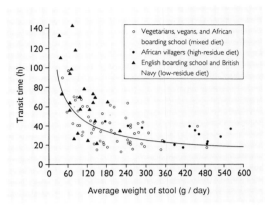

Figure 3.1 Relationship of fibre intake, transit time, and stool weight.

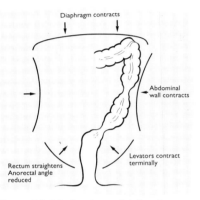

Figure 3.2 Mechanisms of defecation

- Faeces enter rectum
- Reflex relaxation of sphincter
- Intra-abdominal pressure rises
- Anorectal angle straightens
- Gut contraction empties left colon into rectum
- Faeces squeezed through anus

Causes of constipation

Anorectal disorders—Anal fissure; anal stenosis; anterior mucosal prolapse; descending perineum syndrome; haemorrhoids; perianal abscess; rectocele; tumours

Colonic disorders—The irritable bowel syndrome; diverticular disease; tumours; strictures: carcinoma, Crohn's disease, diverticulitis, ulcerative colitis, ischaemic colitis, tuberculosis, amoebiasis, syphilis, lymphogranuloma venereum, endometriosis; hernias; volvulus; intussusception; ulcerative colitis with right sided faecal stasis; pneumatosis cystoides intestinalis; idiopathic slow transit constipation

Pelvic causes—Pregnancy and the puerperium; ovarian and uterine tumours; endometriosis

Neuromuscular causes—*Peripheral:* Hirschsprung's disease, autonomic neuropathy, Chagas' disease, intestinal pseudo-obstruction; *central:* cerebrovascular accident, cerebral tumours, Parkinson's disease, meningocele, multiple sclerosis, tabes dorsalis, paraplegia,

cauda equina tumour, trauma to lumbosacral cord or cauda equina, Shy–Dragar syndrome; *muscular:* dermatomyositis, dystrophia myotonica, progressive systemic sclerosis

Psychiatric disorders—Depression; anorexia nervosa; denied bowel action

Endocrine—Diabetes mellitus; hypercalcaemia; hypothyroidism; hypopituitarism; phaeochromocytoma

Metabolic—Hypokalaemia; lead poisoning; porphyria; uraemia

Environmental—Debility; dehydration; immobilisation; use of bed pan

Drug induced—Anaesthetics; analgesics; antacids (containing aluminium and calcium); anticholinergics; anticonvulsants; antidepressives; antihypertensives; antiparkinsonian drugs; diuretics; ganglion blocking drugs; iron; laxatives (habitual abuse); monoamine oxidase inhibitors; oral contraceptives; psychotherapeutic agents

9A barium enema examination should be performed in all patients in whom constipation is of acute onset as an underlying organic disorder is likely. Strictures require assessment by colonoscopy and biopsy to determine whether the cause is inflammatory or neoplastic. Commonly, however, the stricture is too narrow to permit passage of the endoscope and laparotomy is required to establish the diagnosis.

Right sided faecal stasis is well recognised in patients with ulcerative colitis and can be diagnosed on plain abdominal radiography and barium enema examination, as can pneumatosis cystoides intestinalis, a condition characterised by the presence of gas filled cysts in the large and small intestines. Idiopathic slow transit constipation occurs mainly in young women; it should be suspected when constipation proves refractory to bulk laxatives and may be confirmed by marker studies.

Constipation commonly occurs in the later stages of pregnancy and the puerperium and it may also be caused by ovarian and uterine tumours. Enquiry about menstruation and its disorders and a pelvic examination should, therefore, be considered in women presenting with constipation.

Hirschsprung's disease is characterised by an aganglionic rectosigmoidal segment with inefficient motility, proximal to which the colon is dilated. Although it usually presents in infancy, it may occasionally present in later life. The condition is diagnosed by the absence of ganglion cells in a full thickness rectal biopsy specimen taken at least 2 cm from the dentate line. Its characteristic clinical features suggest autonomic neuropathy, which should prompt formal tests of autonomic function.

Intestinal pseudo-obstruction is characterised by symptoms of recurrent intestinal obstruction in the absence of any evidence of mechanical obstruction. Typically, dilated loops of small and large intestine are seen in plain abdominal radiographs or barium radiographs. This condition may be primary or occur secondary to a number of causes. Studies of intestinal motility may be useful in diagnosis.

Some patients, usually young women, report not having a bowel action for a week or more. Endocrine and metabolic disorders may be suspected clinically and confirmed biochemically. Debility and dehydration may be seen in patients in the community and in hospital patients. Admission to hospital may also lead to constipation through immobilisation and use of bed pans.

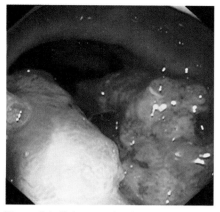

Figure 3.3 Colonoscopic view of a carcinoma of the colon.

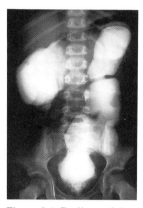

Figure 3.4 Radiograph in patient with Hirschsprung's disease shows a megacolon.

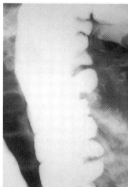

Figure 3.5 Intestinal pseudoobstruction in scleroderma. Radiograph of barium enema examination shows megacolon.

Dietary fibre in common foods (g/kg)

Flour		Vegetables		Swedes	28
Bran	440	(Boiled unless stated)		Sweetcorn (tinned)	57
Brown	75	Baked beans (tinned)	73	Turnips	22
White	30	Beans—broad	42		
Wholemeal	96	Beans—french	32	Fruits	
		Beetroot	25	Apples (peeled)	20
Bread		Brussel sprouts	29	Apricots (dried)	240
Brown	51	Cabbage	25	Bananas	34
White	27	Carrots	31	Figs (dried)	185
Wholemeal	85	Cauliflower	18	Oranges	20
		Celery	22	Peaches	14
Cereals		Parsnips	25	Pears	17
Cornflakes	110	Peas (frozen)	120	Prunes (dried)	161
Muesli	74	Potatoes			
Porridge	8	baked/old	25	Nuts	
Puffed Wheat	154	boiled/new	20	Almonds	143
Shredded Wheat	123	chips/frozen/fried	32	Coconut (Desiccated)	235
		Spinach	63	Peanuts	81

Treatment

General measures

The first consideration in the treatment of patients with constipation is carefully to define the presenting symptoms. If the problem is straining at passing stools, is it painless or painful? If it is painless simple advice about increasing the fibre content of the diet, such as by eating more fruit and vegetables, may suffice and further assessment is not indicated. If, however, the problem is painful constipation this is likely to be part of the irritable bowel syndrome. In patients with constipation induced by general causes, such as lack of exercise, ignoring the need to pass stools, irregular meals, shift work, and poor toilet facilities, sometimes the recognition and correction of these causes are all that is required.

Laxatives

Laxatives are classified into; bulking agents, which include dietary fibre and the bulk laxatives; contact cathartics; stool softeners; osmotic laxatives; and rectal evacuants. When prescribed, the smallest effective dose of laxative should be used. If the bowels become regular, every effort should be made gradually to reduce this dosage.

Megacolon and megarectum may occur due to organic lesions such as Hirschsprung's disease but are most commonly caused by idiopathic constipation. Faecal incontinence caused by impaction with overflow ensues. Enemas may be necessary to empty the colon before attempted retraining of the bowel.

Faecal impaction, which is a particular hazard in elderly people, should ideally be prevented. This can be achieved by checking that patients open their bowels regularly and by giving prophylactic laxatives. In patients with established impaction enemas may be effective but, if not, manual disimpaction should not be unduly delayed.

Refractory constipation

In a few patients constipation proves to be refractory to treatment with a high fibre diet and laxatives. Such patients should be carefully re-evaluated to search for an underlying cause. Plain abdominal radiography and double contrast barium enema examination are mandatory. If these show that the haustral pattern is preserved, and the length and diameter of the large bowel are normal, then it is reasonable to prescribe a more intensive laxative regimen in the first instance. It is sometimes helpful to admit the patient to hospital in order to empty the large bowel by using oral sodium picosulphate or mannitol. This offers the best chance of oral laxatives helping to establish a regular bowel habit. If, however, such measures are ineffective further assessment of colorectal function is indicated.

Hirschprung's disease

Laxatives are unlikely to be effective if the haustral pattern is absent or if there is a megacolon or megarectum. With both Hirschsprung's disease and idiopathic constipation symptoms are usually present from childhood. Anorectal manometry may be helpful in diagnosis because virtually all patients with Hirschsprung's disease have an absent rectosphincteric reflex—that is, the anal sphincter fails to relax when the rectum is distended with a balloon. An absent reflex is, however, occasionally observed in patients with idiopathic constipation. Therefore, in patients with megacolon and an absent reflex a full thickness rectal biopsy is required to distinguish the two conditions.

Laxatives prescribable in the NHS

Bulk forming drugs
Ispaghula husk
Methylcellulose
Sterculia

Stimulant (contact) laxatives
Bisacodyl tablets
Castor oil
Danthron
Docusate sodium (dioctyl sodium sulphosuccinate)
Senna
Sodium picosulphate

Faecal softeners
Liquid paraffin mixture

Osmotic laxatives
Lactulose
Magnesium hydroxide
Magnesium sulphate

Rectally administered laxatives
Bisacodyl suppositories
Glycerol suppositories
Dulco-Lax (bisacodyl)
Phosphate enemas
Beogex (sodium add phosphate) suppositories
Dioctyl
Fletchers' retention enemas
Fletchers' Enemettte (docusate sodium, glycerol, macrogol, sorbic acid)
Klyx enema (docusate sodium, sorbitol)
Microenemas (sodium citrate and other agents)
Veripaque (oxyphenisatin) enemas

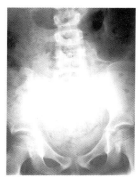

Figure 3.6 Constipation in a child.

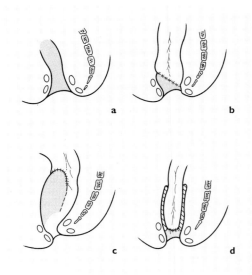

Figure 3.7 Abdominoperineal surgical procedures most commonly used in management of Hirschsprung's disease. (a) Before surgery (stippled area represents aganglionic bowel); (b) rectosigmoidectomy; (c) retrorectal transcolonic pull through; (d) endorectal pull through with primary anastomosis.

Treatment—The treatment of Hirschsprung's disease is surgical. In short segment disease anorectal myectomy, rectal myectomy, or anal sphincterotomy may effect a cure. A diseased distal segment may be bypassed by various pull through procedures. Alternatively, extensive colonic resection with preservation of the diseased segment may produce a more fluid passage of stools and alleviate symptoms.

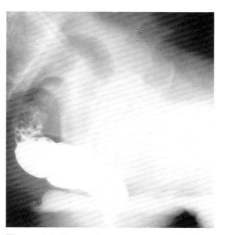

Figure 3.8 Defecating proctogram showing perineal descent.

Severe idiopathic constipation

Research on colorectal function in patients with severe idiopathic constipation has revealed several pathophysiological derangements that are common in this group of conditions. The anorectal angle during attempted defecation was reduced in some, who were unable to evacuate a balloon containing barium from the rectum. Electromyography of the pelvic floor may show increased puborectalis activity on attempted defecation. This leads to a functional rectal stenosis and constipation caused by anorectal spasm.

Whole gut transit time is often delayed. The other recognised abnormality in motor function is failure of the pelvic floor to relax on attempted defecation—the outlet syndrome. This may be diagnosed by balloon proctography or electromyography. Electromyography may identify pudendal neuropathy in patients with perineal descent and chronic straining at passing stools. Perineal descent can be shown radiologically by screening of a barium filled rectum during straining. It may cause recurrent trauma to the pudendal nerves leading to denervation and weakness of the external anal sphincter. Patients remain constipated because they have an abnormal, counterproductive increase in activity in both the external anal sphincter and puborectalis on straining and thus maintain the anorectal angle despite bulging the perineum.

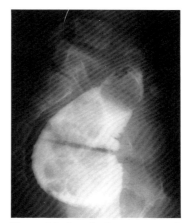

Figure 3.9 Acquired megarectum loaded with faeces.

Treatment—(1) Behaviour therapy, biofeedback, psychotherapy: biofeedback has been successfully used in the management of idiopathic constipation and faecal soiling in children and adolescents. By learning to control sphincter activity children have been able to establish a regular bowel habit. Behaviour therapy and psychotherapy may also prove helpful in the treatment of constipation. (2) Surgery: anorectal myectomy may prove effective in the treatment of the outlet syndrome. This operation is contraindicated, however, when marker studies indicate severe colonic inertia. The results of myectomy are also poor in those who develop constipation after the age of 10. Such patients may benefit from a total colectomy and ileorectal anastomosis. This operation may also be of benefit in patients with severe idiopathic slow transit constipation. However, the precise role of surgery in the treatment of refractory constipation awaits definition.

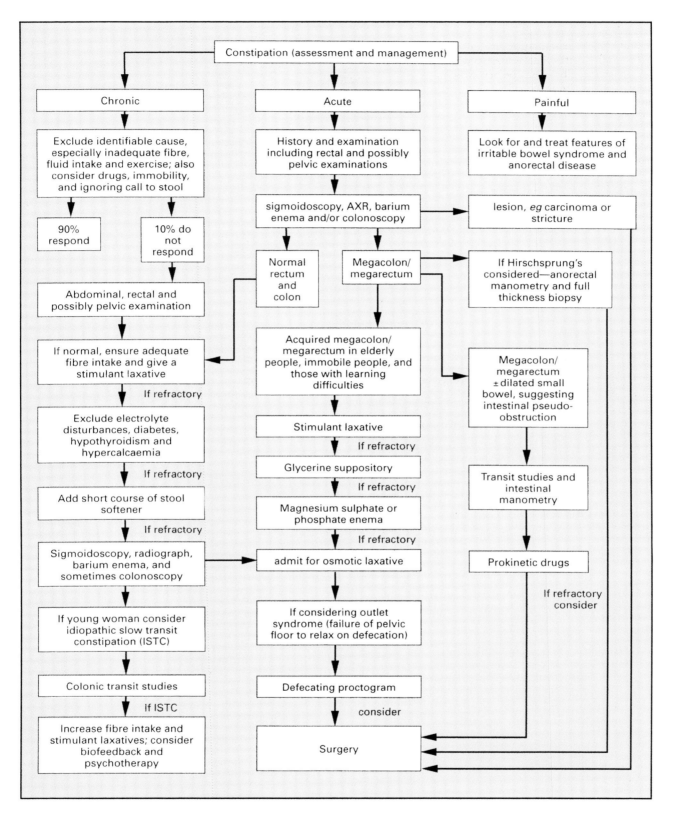

Figure 3.10 Assessment and management of constipation.

Conclusions

The assessment of patients with constipation depends on a careful consideration of the possible causes combined with a detailed history and clinical examination, including sigmoidoscopy. Treatment with dietary fibre and bulk laxatives is usually effective. These may be beneficial in various colorectal disorders such as simple constipation, diverticular disease, and the irritable bowel syndrome.

If treatment is ineffective, barium enema examination and sometimes colonoscopy are required. These investigations are indicated in the first instance in older patients presenting with constipation and in any patient with constipation of sudden onset. In patients with refractory constipation specialised investigations of anal and colorectal function are indicated to identify conditions such as Hirschsprung's disease and various abnormalities in severe idiopathic constipation. The treatment of Hirschsprung's disease is surgical. Surgery may also help some patients with severe idiopathic constipation, although behavioural management and psychotherapy may also be effective.

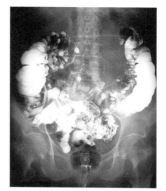

Figure 3.11 Diverticular disease on barium enema examination.

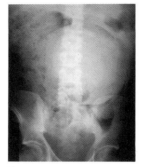

Figure 3.12 Chronic constipation: radiograph shows a huge faecal mass.

The graph is reproduced with permission of *The Lancet* (from Burkitt *et al*, 1972;**ii**:1408–12). We thank the staff of the medical illustration departments of Bolton General and Hope Hospitals, Dr R Bissett, Miss C Doig, Dr P Strong, and Professor L A Turnberg for preparing and supplying the photographs, and Dr S Wells and Norgine Ltd for information.

4 Diarrhoea

A J M Watson

Diarrhoea can be defined as the passage of more than three loose stools a day. This results from an increase in the stool water content. In hospital practice, diarrhoea can be more accurately defined as an increase in stool weight or volume (>200 g).

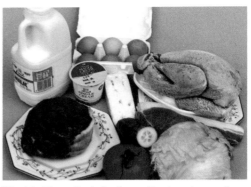

Fig 4.1 Many foods harbour diarrhoeal organisms.

History and examination

History

Diarrhoea should be distinguished from faecal incontinence with normal stool volume and frequency, the passage of blood and mucus, and the frequent passage of a small volume of stool, as can occur in patients with the irritable bowel syndrome. In disease of the distal colon or rectum there is usually frequent passage of small quantities of dark stool, often with urgency. The presence of *visible* blood usually implies colonic disease. Pain is in the left lower quadrant, is relieved by defecation, and may be associated with tenesmus. In disease of the small bowel or proximal colon, the stools are of large volume and watery or, if there is steatorrhoea, pale and offensive. Pain, if present, is periumbilical or in the right lower quadrant.

If the diarrhoea is acute (lasts for less than three weeks), infective causes are likely and corroborating evidence should be sought, such as travel abroad, ingestion of raw seafood, and concomitant diarrhoea in family members and close contacts (Table 4.1). The irritable bowel syndrome, ulcerative colitis, and Crohn's disease are the most common causes of chronic diarrhoea in the United Kingdom. A careful history usually shows that patients with the irritable bowel syndrome suffer from frequent passage of small volumes of stool rather than "true" diarrhoea as defined above. Symptoms have often been present for many years without evidence of serious organic disease. However, care should be taken in diagnosing the irritable bowel syndrome in middle aged or elderly patients because serious organic disease can be missed. If there is a change of bowel habit (constipation alternating with

Table 4.1 Symptoms and signs associated with chronic diarrhoea

Symptom or sign	Chronic diarrhoeal syndrome
Arthritis	Ulcerative colitis, Crohn's disease, Whipple's disease
Liver disease	Ulcerative colitis, Crohn's disease, colonic cancer with metastases
Fever	Ulcerative colitis, Crohn's disease, amoebiasis, Whipple's disease, tuberculosis
Neuropathy	Diabetic diarrhoea, amyloidosis
Severe weight loss	Malabsorption, cancer, thyrotoxicosis, inflammatory bowel disease
Lymphadenopathy	Lymphoma, AIDS, Whipple's disease
Uveitis	Ulcerative colitis, Crohn's disease
Erythema nodosum	Inflammatory bowel disease, yersiniosis
Dermatitis herpetiformis	Coeliac disease
Flushing	Carcinoid syndrome
Pyoderma gangrenosum	Ulcerative colitis

Table 4.2 Common bacterial and protozoal causes of acute' diarrhoea in the United Kingdom and their sources

Bacteria	Food source	Symptoms	Incubation period
Salmonella spp.	Eggs, poultry, beef, milk, salads	Slimy "pea soup" stools, fever	6–24 h
Campylobacter spp.	Poultry, milk	Bloody diarrhoea, abdominal pain, fever, generalised malaise, coryza, headache	48–72 h
Clostridium perfringens	Poultry, beef	Watery diarrhoea, abdominal pain	8–24 h
Staphylococcus aureus	Poultry, salads	Diarrhoea, vomiting	2–6 h
Shigella spp.	Salads	Diarrhoea initially watery becoming bloody later, fever	36–48 h
Bacillus cereus	Fried rice	Diarrhoea, abdominal pain, vomiting	1–6 h
Giardia lamblia	Water, person to person contact, homosexual contact	Diarrhoea, steatorrhoea	7–14 days

diarrhoea), particularly in a patient over 50, it is mandatory to exclude colon cancer. A drug history is also important because some frequently prescribed drugs can cause diarrhoea (for example, propranolol, methyldopa, theophylline, frusemide, and ampicillin).

Examination

The main objective of examination of patients with acute diarrhoea is to determine the severity of dehydration and electrolyte depletion. Fever suggests infection with *Salmonella*, *Shigella*, or *Campylobacter* species. A rectal examination and sigmoidoscopy should be performed, both to assess the degree of rectal inflammation if present and to obtain faeces for analysis. Some signs of specific chronic diarrhoeal diseases are listed in Table 4.2.

Investigation

In acute diarrhoea investigations should be concentrated initially on identification of possible infective agents. In patients with chronic diarrhoea sigmoidoscopy and rectal biopsy are mandatory to assess mucosal inflammation, tumours and the presence of melanosis coli, which might indicate laxative abuse. Figure 4.3 outlines the investigation of diarrhoea.

Useful simple tests

Stool volume—This is a useful part of the assessment of diarrhoea and monitoring its treatment in hospital. (Note that the mass of stools in grams is equivalent to their volume in millilitres. If the stools cannot be weighed immediately they can be frozen.) In the UK, high volume stool output (>800 ml/24 h) without inflammation of the bowel is most commonly caused by laxative abuse.

Stool electrolytes—In cases of large volume watery diarrhoea measurement of stool electrolytes and osmolality can be helpful. The total stool ion concentration can be estimated as $2 \times (Na^+ + K^+)$. If the measured stool osmolality is more than 50 mmol/l greater than the estimated total ion content, then the diarrhoea is likely to be caused by the presence of a non-absorbed solute. In adult practice in the United Kingdom, this is usually a laxative such as lactulose or a magnesium salt. Deficiency of brush border lactase is both uncommon and usually does not cause symptoms even when present. If the two values are similar then the diarrhoea is likely to be secretory.

Stool alkalinisation—An important, though uncommon, cause of chronic watery diarrhoea is purgative abuse. Phenolphthalein ingestion can sometimes be identified by the addition of 1 drop of molar NaOH to 3 ml of stool water. This is, however, an insensitive technique and cannot detect bisacodyl, senna derived laxatives, or danthron. Chromatography of urine is highly sensitive and specific, and is the analytical method of choice. If not available locally, samples should be sent to a laboratory elsewhere with experience of this type of analysis.

Treatment

The treatment of diarrhoea will depend on the cause. Some general principles are discussed below.

Rehydration

The importance of rehydration must be emphasised. In the United Kingdom there is still an appreciable mortality from diarrhoeal disease in infants and elderly people because of inadequate rehydration. A postural drop in diastolic blood pressure of >20 mm Hg or a rise in pulse of >20 beats/minute or fever of >38·5°C together with severe abdominal pain are

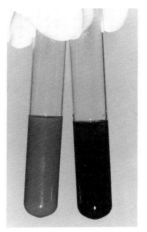

Figure 4.2 Normal stools (left) and stools after misuse of purgatives (right). Alkalinisation of phenolphthalein laxatives in the stool with sodium hydroxide causes a colour change.

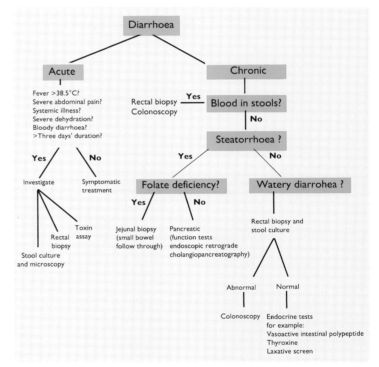

Figure 4.3 Flow diagram showing the investigation of diarrhoea.

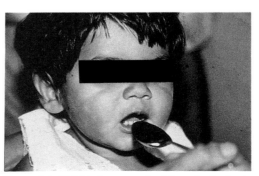

Figure 4.4 Child being treated with oral rehydration solution.

15

signs of severe disease. In such cases treatment with intravenous fluids in hospital is mandatory. In milder cases rehydration should be with oral rehydration fluids. Usually this can be achieved adequately at home.

The optimal formulation of oral rehydration fluids is still debated but a sodium ion concentration of 50–70 mmol/l (Rehidrat, Electrolade) is probably best for United Kingdom practice. The recommended sodium ion concentration in the *British National Formulary* is probably too low (35–60 mmol/l) whereas that recommended by the World Health Organization is too high (90 mmol/l) and more appropriate for practice in the developing countries where sodium ion depletion is common. With young children sips of the fluid (5–10 ml) should be given every 10 minutes. Research has shown that, despite vomiting adequate rehydration can be achieved if it is administered this way.

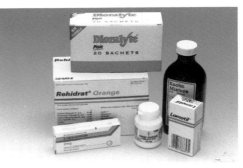

Figure 4.5 Some popular antidiarrhoeal drugs.

Antibiotic treatment

Antibiotics are not usually indicated for diarrhoea. In the United Kingdom most acute infective diarrhoeal illnesses are caused by viruses. Of the common causative bacteria only certain *Shigella* spp. and *Campylobacter jejuni* can be treated with antibiotics, but this is indicated only in severe cases. Infection with *Shigella sonnei*, which is the most common causative species in the United Kingdom, does not require antibiotic treatment. Infection with other *Shigella* spp. can be treated with ampicillin 50–100 mg/kg in children or 2 g daily in adults. Erythromycin is effective against *C. jejuni* if patients start taking it early in the course of the disease. In most cases of gastroenteritis caused by *Salmonella* species antibiotics are not given. Exceptions include patients with immunosuppression, patients with malignancies, babies, very old people, and patients with severe sepsis. In such cases ampicillin, trimethoprim, or ciprofloxacin can be given. *Clostridium difficile* causes pseudomembranous colitis, and this usually occurs in patients in hospital after treatment with antibiotics. The disease should be treated with metronidazole or vancomycin only if it is severe and symptomatic. Giardiasis is treated with metronidazole (2 g for three days).

Traveller's diarrhoea—Traveller's diarrhoea is caused principally by enterotoxogenic *Escherichia coli* (40–75% of cases). It is treated with trimethoprim 200 mg three times daily for three days, along with vigorous hydration. Prophylaxis with trimethoprim, while effective, may cause the emergence of resistant strains. In any case, traveller's diarrhoea, once contracted, can be controlled rapidly with trimethoprim and an antimotility agent. If patients are given antibiotics before going abroad, they should be counselled on the indications for self administration of antibiotics and told to seek medical advice if the diarrhoea is bloody, associated with a fever of >38·5°C, or associated with severe abdominal pain.

Symptomatic treatment

Antimotility agents such as loperamide (Imodium), diphenoxylate (Lomotil), and codeine are effective for treating symptoms. They are contraindicated in acute infective diarrhoea with bloody stools as they will slow the clearance of infective agents. They can, however, be helpful in ulcerative colitis and Crohn's disease, although they should be used with caution in severe exacerbations as toxic dilatation can be induced.

Indications for antibiotic treatment

- Severe cases of infection with *Shigella* spp. and *Campylobacter jejuni*
  For *Shigella* spp. other than *S. sonnei* give ciprofloxin in adults and ampicillin in children
  For *C. jejuni* give erythromycin in severe cases
- Immunosuppressed patients, babies, and very old people infected with *Salmonella* spp.—give ampicillin, trimethoprim, or ciprofloxacin
- Severe cases of infection with *Clostridium difficile*—give vancomycin or metronidazole
- Giardiasis—give metronidazole 2 g · for three days

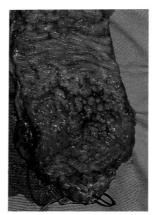

Figure 4.6 Resected rectum from a patient with severe proctocolitis who had suffered longstanding profuse diarrhoea.

5 Lower gastrointestinal haemorrhage

D J Jones

Bleeding from the lower gastrointestinal tract is a common clinical problem in both general and hospital practice. Patients are alarmed when they pass blood, but most have minor anorectal disorders that can be investigated and treated on an outpatient or day case basis. A smaller proportion have colorectal neoplasia, inflammatory bowel disease, or profuse life threatening haemorrhage. Lower gastrointestinal haemorrhage affects people of all ages, though the aetiology varies in different age groups.

Common clinical patterns of bleeding

The character of blood lost is dependent on the rate of haemorrhage and the site of the source. Patients with brisk haemorrhage and those with distal colorectal lesions tend to pass bright red blood. If the bleeding is slow or the source is in the proximal colon the blood is altered, being darker red in colour, and mixed with faeces.

Haemorrhoids—Patients with bleeding haemorrhoids pass bright red streaks of blood, which they initially notice on the faeces, on toilet tissue, or in the toilet bowl. Occasionally bleeding can be vigorous and actually drip from the anal canal. Such bleeding is usually associated with large or prolapsed haemorrhoids and can occur spontaneously.

Inflammatory bowel disease—Patients with inflammatory bowel disease tend to lose small amounts of blood mixed with mucus and faeces and they usually have increased bowel frequency. Similar symptoms are also seen in patients with irradiation proctocolitis, which usually follows radiotherapy for pelvic malignancy.

Tumours—Patients with distal colorectal polyps and cancers pass bright red or slightly altered streaks of blood, and this is a common presenting symptom. If the tumour is in the proximal colon the blood lost is darker in colour, and less obvious. Patients with caecal cancer commonly present with iron deficiency anaemia caused by occult chronic blood loss with apparently normal unaltered faeces.

Diverticular disease and angiodysplasia—Bleeding in patients with colonic diverticular disease and colonic angiodysplasia is often brisk, causing a sudden urge to defecate, followed by the passage of a large dark red stool. This may be repeated but the bleeding usually stops spontaneously. The bleeding may be sufficient to cause life threatening hypovolaemic shock. Severe haemorrhage occasionally develops in patients with solitary rectal ulcers.

Ischaemic colitis—Patients with ischaemic colitis are usually elderly and present with left sided abdominal pain associated with blood stained diarrhoea.

Management of minor bleeding

Most patients with minor bleeding can be investigated and treated as outpatients. Anorectal examination, sigmoidoscopy, colonoscopy, and barium enema examination form the mainstay of diagnosis, and the disorder is usually easily identified and treated appropriately. Haemorrhoids are extremely common and should not be assumed to be the cause of bleeding until more serious conditions such as neoplasia and inflammatory bowel disease have been excluded.

Causes of lower gastrointestinal haemorrhage

Children
Meckel's diverticulum
Juvenile polyps
Inflammatory bowel disease

Adults
Inflammatory bowel disease
Adenomatous polyps
Carcinoma
Arteriovenous malformations
Small intestinal neoplasia
Hereditary telangiectasia
Infective colitis
Haemorrhoids
Solitary rectal ulcer
Anal fissure

Elderly people
Diverticular disease
Angiodysplasia
Adenomatous polyps
Carcinoma
Ischaemic colitis
Inflammatory bowel disease
Radiation proctitis

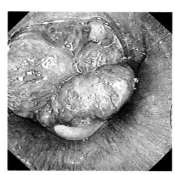

Figure 5.1 Haemorrhoids viewed through a proctoscope

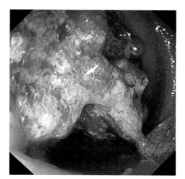

Figure 5.2 Endoscopic view of a carcinoma of the sigmoid colon.

Management of minor lower gastrointestinal haemorrhage

- History and general examination
- Anorectal examination
- Proctosigmoidoscopy
- Colonoscopy
- Double contrast barium enema examination
- Treatment of cause

Major lower gastrointestinal bleeding

Patients with recurrent or profuse bleeding pose a diagnostic dilemma because the source of their haemorrhage is notoriously difficult to identify. Ninety per cent of them have either colonic angiodysplasia or diverticular disease.

Diverticular disease

Traditionally, diverticular disease was considered to be the most common cause of major lower gastrointestinal haemorrhage. Bleeding occurs when a blood vessel breaks down, as it passes through the weakened wall of a diverticulum in a submucuous plane. Diverticular disease is a common finding on barium enema examination and for this reason has been implicated as the source of bleeding in the absence of any other discernible abnormality. Many cases of lower gastrointestinal bleeding that would previously have been attributred to diverticular disease are now recognised as resulting from colonic angiodysplasia.

Angiodysplasia

Colonic angiodysplasia is an acquired condition, predominantly affecting the elderly. The lesions are small vascular swellings, usually less than 5 mm in diameter, comprising dilated venules located immediately beneath the mucosa. They can be shown by colonoscopy and arteriography but are easily overlooked, and techniques such as injecting the blood vessels of resected specimens with silicone rubber solutions and barium have been used to identify and confirm their presence. Most lesions are located in the right colon and they are often multiple. Angiodysplasia may also affect the small bowel. Colonic angiodysplasia often coexist with other abnormalities that have haemorrhagic potential, such as a Meckel's diverticulum, which may cause confusion in determining the true source of bleeding. Many patients also have associated cardiovascular disorders.

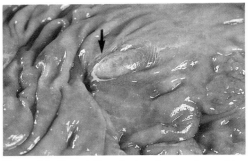

Figure 5.3 Caecal diverticulum in a patient with colonic bleeding. Barium has been injected into the blood vessels after resection to show the site of bleeding—it can be seen extravasating from the diverticulum (arrow).

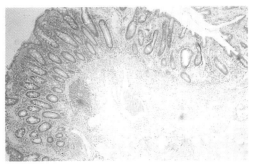

Figure 5.4 Photomicrograph showing dilated submucosal venule of a colonic angiodysplasia.

Management of major haemorrhage

A patient with major haemorrhage is resuscitated, a baseline red blood cell count and packed cell volume determined, blood cross matched, and a coagulopathy excluded. Gastroscopy should be performed to be certain that the patient does not have upper gastrointestinal haemorrhage, as the colour of blood passed may be misleading. Anorectal examination, proctoscopy, and sigmoidoscopy should be performed to identify the occasional haemorrhoid, carcinoma, and severe proctocolitis, which bleed profusely. But the source of bleeding is not usually disclosed by these investigations. Colonoscopy is usually unrewarding during active bleeding as the mucosa is obscured by bloody faeces.

In most patients the bleeding stops spontaneously or slows down, providing an opportunity to perform a more rewarding colonoscopy with the aid of good suction and insufflaton. If abnormalities such as polyps or angiodysplasia are discovered, biopsy specimens can be taken or they can be treated endoscopically by snaring, electrocoagulation, or laser treatment. A barium enema examination will not give useful information during an acute bleeding episode and barium lying in the colon will interfere with the interpretation of arteriograms, which may be subsequently indicated. A double contrast barium enema radiograph after the acute haemorrhage has resolved may provide useful information, but colonoscopy offers greater diagnostic and therapeutic potential.

Management of major lower gastrointestinal haemorrhage
- Resuscitaton
- History
- Anorectal examination
- Proctosigmoidoscopy
- Colonoscopy (endoscopic treatment)
- Isotope scanning or arteriography (if the bleeding continues)
- Laparotomy; on table endoscopy
- Resection

Identifying the source of haemorrhage not revealed by endoscopy
- Isotope red cell scan
- Selective arteriography
- Small bowel endoscopy

Identifying the source

The most useful investigations for profuse or continuing bleeding not identified by an endoscopic technique are scanning with red blood cells labelled with technetium-99m, sulphur colloid isotope scanning, and selective mesenteric arteriography. Isotope scanning is the most sensitive and will show extravasation into the gut with bleeding of the order of 0·05–0·1 ml/min. The precise anatomical localisation of the lesion may, however, be difficult to determine, and repeated images taken over several hours may be needed to follow the path of extravasated red cells through the bowel to localise the source. Selective arteriography of the inferior and superior mesenteric arteries and coeliac axis will identify the anatomical site of bleeding more accurately, but the technique is invasive and successful only if the bleeding is brisk, in the order of 1 ml/min.

An occasional vascular abnormality may be shown in the absence of profuse bleeding. Some vascular abnormalities can be treated by embolisation at the time of arteriography or a local infusion of vasopressin may be administered, though these treatments are not widely practised at present.

Surgery for major haemorrhage

If haemorrhage continues and the bleeding cannot be controlled endoscopically, surgery is indicated. If the bleeding lesion has been accurately localised before surgery, an appropriate segmental resection can be confidently performed. If the source cannot be shown, surgery may still be necessary to control haemorrhage and should be considered in patients requiring a blood transfusion of 4 units or more within 24 hours.

The entire bowel is carefully palpated and some lesions such as small bowel tumours may be immediately obvious. Commonly the source is not apparent and the location of blood within the bowel can be misleading. There is a lack of unanimity regarding the preferred procedure for these patients. The most common site of such bleeding is caecal angiodysplasia and this knowledge has been used to justify an empirical right hemicolectomy. This usually controls the haemorrhage, but a minority of patients with a lesion elsewhere in the colon may rebleed and require a further operation and resection, which carries an increased risk of morbidity and mortality.

On table lavage of the bowel and intraoperative colonoscopy may help identify the source of bleeding if the patient's condition is stable. This is facilitated by operating on all patients with lower gastrointestinal haemorrhage with their legs raised in supports. A catheter is introduced through a small caecostomy or the base of a removed appendix and warm saline infused to clean the colon. A colonoscope is then introduced through the anus until the point of bleeding is identified, enabling an appropriate segmental colectomy to be performed. This is a time consuming procedure which is often unsuccessful and unsuitable for unstable patients.

An alternative strategy is to perform a subtotal colectomy with ileorectal anastomosis. In experienced hands this does not take much longer than a segmental resection and rebleeding is rarely a problem. The disadvantage is the increased frequency of defecation, which can be particularly troublesome in elderly patients, whose continence may already be compromised. Some patients who are found to have probable angiodysplastic lesions on isotope scanning or arteriography subsequently stop bleeding. These patients do not require immediate surgery but can be subject to a policy of active observation. Patients who present with a major haemorrhage carry a high risk of futher haemorrhage. If their angiodysplasia can be visualised on

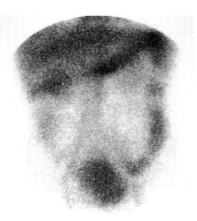

Figure 5.5 Isotope labelled red blood cell scan in a patient with caecal angiodysplasia, showing extravasation into the caecum, which has then outlined the colon.

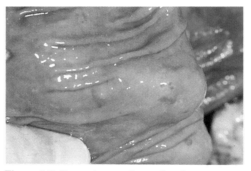

Figure 5.6 Operative specimen showing angiodysplasia, which was the cause of bleeding.

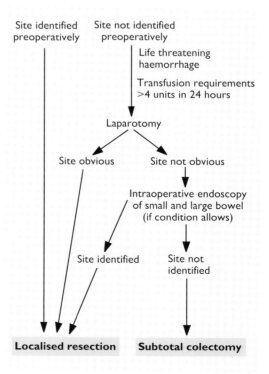

Figure 5.7 Flow chart for surgery for major gastrointestinal haemorrhage not responding to conservative or endoscopic treatment.

subsequent colonoscopy they can be treated endoscopically. Alternatively, they should be offered early elective resection if their general condition permits.

Ischaemic colitis

Ischaemic colitis is characterised by a fairly sudden onset of left sided abdominal pain associated with bloody diarrhoea and left sided abdominal tenderness. Most cases can occur spontaneously but it is also seen in a small number of patients after aortic surgery. Some patients have evidence of occlusive atheromatous disease or embolism affecting the inferior mesenteric artery. Patients with less severe arteriosclerotic disease may develop ischaemic colitis after a period of hypotension or cardiac failure. Most patients are elderly and many have coexistent cardiorespiratory problems. A large number of patients with ischaemic colitis do not have any evidence of significant mesenteric vascular disease and their disorder is of uncertain aetiology.

Ischaemic colitis predominantly affects the mucosa, which undergoes necrosis and ulceration, and only rarely does it progress to complete ischaemia and gangrene of the colon. Most patients' condition resolves spontaneously but about a half proceed to develop a fibrous stricture. The splenic flexture, descending colon, and sigmoid colon are the most commonly involved sites.

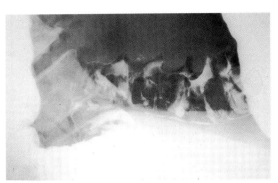

Figure 5.8 Contrast study showing characteristic "thumb printing" indicative of ulceration in a patient with ischaemic colitis.

Diagnosis

A high index of suspicion is required to reach the diagnosis. Sigmoidoscopy reveals a normal rectal mucosa, with blood stained liquid faeces coming from the more proximal colon. Careful colonoscopy with minimal insufflation will reach the involved segment, which appears ulcerated and haemorrhagic. Biopsy specimens usually show non-specific inflammatory changes. A barium enema examination performed during the acute phase will show characteristics "thumb printing", reflecting mucosal oedema and ulceration.

Management

Patients are managed conservatively with supportive treatment and active observation. Most settle and should be followed up with further barium studies to identify those who develop strictures. Surgery is indicated in patients who develop signs of peritonitis. Those with gangrene usually present with signs of an intra-abdominal catastrophe and the diagnosis is usually made at laparotomy. These patients have a high mortality (>50%). The involved bowel is resected and the ends either exteriorised or anastomosed, depending on the circumstances.

Management of ischaemic colitis	
Symptoms	*Treatment*
Mild symptoms No evidence of peritonitis or perforation	Active observation
Peritonitis, frank gangrene	Urgent colectomy

Irradiation proctitis

Irradiation proctitis is an occasional cause of bleeding in patients who have received abdominal or pelvic radiotherapy, usually for cancers of the bladder or of the female genital tract. An obliterative arteritis develops in the irradiated large bowel. This causes mucosal ischaemia, ulceration, and bleeding. Patients have symptoms similar to those of inflammatory bowel disease, which may appear and progress several years after the radiotherapy. Chronic blood loss may lead to anaemia necessitating transfusion. In severe cases a rectovaginal fistula may develop. Topical steroid enemas may be prescribed, but irradiation proctitis is usually resistant to medical treatment. Diversionary stomas may ease the blood loss temporarily but the condition usually progresses. For severe symptoms and persistent blood loss, resection of the diseased rectum is indicated with either a coloanal anastomosis or a permanent colostomy depending on the extent of the disease.

Management of irradiation proctitis

Minor symptoms
- No treatment
- Trial of topical steroids

Severe symptoms
- Rectal excision
- Coloanal anastomosis or abdominoperineal excision and colostomy

6 The irritable bowel syndrome

K J Moriarty

Patients with the irritable bowel syndrome can be subdivided into those with spastic constipation, who have abdominal pain related to disturbances of bowel action, and those with painless diarrhoea, who complain of increased stool frequency not associated with abdominal pain.

Most patients with the syndrome have "functional abdominal pain". As this may arise at any site from the oesophagus to the rectum the expression "irritable gut" may be more appropriate. The expression "functional pain" is sometimes used inappropriately to suggest that the pain does not really exist or "is in the patient's mind". Functional pain can, however, be just as severe and disabling as organic pain.

About 30% of people with functional gastrointestinal symptoms such as abdominal pain, erratic bowel habit, and abdominal distension have the irritable bowel syndrome diagnosed.

Gastrointestinal symptoms and disorders in the irritable bowel syndrome

Halitosis; unpleasant taste; dry mouth; ptyalism; furred tongue; burning tongue; lump in the throat; globus sensation; chronic or recurrent nausea; psychogenic vomiting; rumination; heartburn; water brash; postprandial epigasric fullness; early satiety; butterflies in the abdomen; sinking feeling in the pit of the abdomen; tachygastria; gas: aerophagia, burping, belching, borborygmus (gurgling), wind, distension, excessive flatus; abdominal bloating; proctalgia fugax; dyschezia; tenesmus; incomplete evacuation; mucus; runny stools, straining: painless, painful

---

Pathophysiology

Psychological factors

The irritable bowel syndrome is commonly associated with psychological or psychiatric disorders, especially anxiety, depression, and neuroses. People with these disorders seem particularly susceptible to developing abdominal pain in response to stress. Stress plays an important part in the pathogenesis of pain. Many patients, however, do not have any obvious psychological or personality disorder.

Motility

Abnormal bursts of motor activity in the colon have been demonstrated in relation to episodes of pain in some patients, and small intestinal and gastric motility derangements have been described in patients with pain. The relationship between motor disturbances and pain is not, however, clear cut.

In patients with spastic constipation an increased frequency and amplitude of segmenting non-propulsive colonic contractions have been observed. This may cause narrowing of a segment of bowel and distension proximal to this area, producing pain. In contrast, decreased colonic motor activity has been recorded in patients with painless diarrhoea. Also, the transit time of a meal through the small bowel of patients with painless diarrhoea is shorter than in those with constipation or pain and distension, highlighing the value of identifying the subgroups of patients with the irritable bowel syndrome, both in facilitating recognition of their pathophysiological derangements and as an aid to providing a rational basis for treatment depending on the patient's symptoms.

Patients with the irritable bowel sysndrome may experience pain throughout the abdomen with referral to extra-abdominal sites. They are abnormally sensitive to distension of the gut by gas or balloons, and trigger areas for pain may be found in the proximal, mid, and distal gut of a patient.

Gastrointestinal infections can lead to the development of the irritable bowel syndrome in susceptible patients. In such patients the disease tends to have a good prognosis.

Associated psychological disorders

Anxiety; depression; neuroses; schizophrenia; anorexia nervosa; hysteria; psychopathy; Münchausen's syndrome

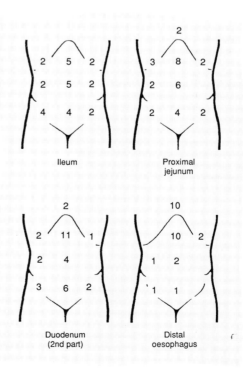

Figure 6.1 Sites of pain on distending a balloon in the gastrointestinal tract of 21 patients. The numbers refer to the number of subjects with pain sited in the positions shown. (From Moriarty and Dawson, *BMJ* 1982;**284**:1670–2.)

Clinical features

The characteristic features of the irritable bowel syndrome are abdominal distension, relief of pain with bowel movement, looser and more frequent bowel movements with the onset of pain, the passage of mucus, and incomplete evacuation. Characteristically the motions are of small volume, are frequent, are pencil-like or similar to rabbits' motions, are often accompanied by urgency, and typically occur in the morning.

Investigative approach

The clinician has a large armamentarium of diagnostic methods by which to identify or exclude organic disease. One approach is to perform a series of endoscopic, barium, and imaging examinations, and to diagnose the irritable bowel syndrome only if all of these yield negative results. Although extensive investigation may sometimes be necessary in difficult cases, this is not recommended. It may be demoralising for the patient, with each investigation that is requested reinforcing the fear of organic disease and each negative result undermining confidence in the doctor's ability to diagnose the source of pain. Moreover, it is not cost effective.

Functional pain is much more common than organic pain and a positive diagnosis can usually be made from the history and clinical examination alone, without the need for extensive investigations. This has the advantage that the early recognition of a functional basis for the patient's pain: expedites the institution of appropriate treatment; minimises the number of investigations and procedures to which the patient is subjected, thereby earning his or her confidence and gratitude; and is cost effective.

Differentiation between organic and functional abdominal pain

Patients with the irritable bowel sydrome often describe a stitch, ache, or discomfort in their abdomen rather than a true pain, and a history of similar attacks over many years, sometimes with long pain free intervals, may be obtained.

Although most commonly felt in the right or left iliac fossa or right hypochondrium, pain of functional origin may be felt anywhere within the abdomen or outside it and tends to be diffuse. Intolerance to fatty foods and flatulence are not, as is commonly thought, clinical features of gall stones but are common in patients with the irritable bowel syndrome. Various non-bowel symptoms are found in patients with the syndrome.

If physical examination, including a rectal examination and sigmoidoscopy, gives normal results further investigation is not usually warranted. At sigmoidoscopy contraction rings may be seen and air insufflation may reproduce the patient's pain, which may reassure both the clinician and the patient. The threshold for investigation should, however, be lower in older patients, especially those over 50 who develop abdominal pains for the first time.

Management

Many patients simply seek explanation and reassurance and to have their fear of organic disease, especially cancer, allayed

---

Discriminating features of a functional gastrointestinal disorder

- Patient's complaints are disproportionate to clinical wellbeing
- Symptoms are unconvincing, or change from time to time
- Patient describes symptoms, especially pain, in dramatic, often bizarre terms
- Symptoms are continuous, occurring daily over long periods of time
- Pain before breakfast but seldom disturbing sleep
- Patient locates or describes pain with sweeping movements of one or both hands
- Pain cannot be relieved
- Morning nausea
- When vomiting occurs the patient cannot eat for several hours afterwards
- History of psychiatric disturbance

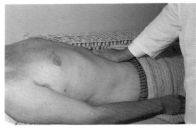

Figure 6.2   Abdominal examination.

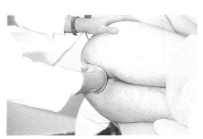

Figure 6.3   Rectal examination.

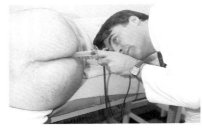

Figure 6.4   Sigmoidoscopy.

Non-colonic features of the irritable bowel syndrome

Nausea/vomiting	Back pain
Dysphagia	Frequent headache
Difficulty finishing meals	Poor sleep
Excessive flatus	Constant tiredness
Dysmenorrhoea	Pruritus
Dyspareunia	Bad breath/unpleasant taste
Urinary frequency	
Urinary urgency	
Urinary hesitancy	
Nocturia	
Incomplete emptying of bladder	

Management of psychological disorders

If anxiety persists despite reassurance and explanation anxiolytic drugs may be indicated for short periods. It is important to recognise and treat depression, which may be masked. Close links between the psychiatrist or psychologist and the gastroenterologist are often helpful in the management of patients with severe irritable bowel syndrome and joint follow up may sometimes be indicated.

Dietary fibre, bran, and bulk laxatives

The prescription of a high fibre diet, bran, or bulk laxatives to a patient with the irritable bowel syndrome may lead to an improvement, deterioration, or no change in the patient's symptoms. A reasonable course is to advise patients taking a low fibre diet to increase their intake of fibre and to adjust this amount according to response, while in those with pain and distension, particularly any who are consuming vast quantities of fibres, a reduced intake may prove beneficial.

Drug therapy

Spasmodic drugs such as dicyclomine and hyoscine butylbromide may be helpful in relieving pain caused by gut spasm, as may the carminative peppermint oil. Antidiarrhoeal agents are of value in patients with frequent stool evacuation, although they may exacerbate abdominal discomfort and constipation in patients with alternating diarrhoea and constipation. If taken at night they may diminish early morning stool frequency. Codeine phosphate, diphenoxylate, and loperamide are generally equally effective.

Although a single drug may help many patients, some require a combination of a laxative or antidiarrhoeal drug with an antispasmodic drug or anxiolytic drug, or both. In combination benefit may be achieved with smaller doses than when these drugs are prescribed alone.

Management of patients with functional abdominal symptoms
All patients
● Make a careful assessment
● Search for psychopathological signs
● Use a sympathetic, interested approach
● Take a history of diet—for example, is it high residue?
● Take a history of smoking, alcohol, stress, and other diseases
● Give reassurance
Some patients
● Give an anxiolytic short term
● Give antidepressants
● Give a bulk laxative
● Give an antidiarrhoeal drug
● Give an antispasmodic
● Perform joint follow up with a psychiatrist or psychologist

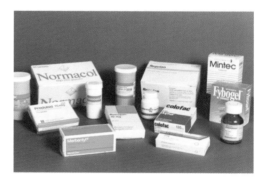

Figure 6.5   Drugs given for the irritable bowel syndrome.

Special problems

Intractable functional abdominal pain

In about 5% of patients pain is refractory to all standard treatment and causes a major disturbance to everyday life. Most of these patients are middle aged women with one or more abdominal scars and vast case notes and *x* ray examination records, usually from several hospitals. The most important aspect of management of these patients is to recognise their problem, accept it, and resist the temptation of extensive and repeated investigation. The clinician can contain the situation by seeing such patients every few months or so and listening sympathetically. Such a policy may help patients to come to terms with their affliction and enhance their ability to cope with it. Hypnotherapy may help in some cases.

Food intolerance

About 75% of patients with the irritable bowel syndrome have pain after eating. This phenomenon of generalised food intolerance must be distinguished from intolerance to specific foods, which may produce symptoms in certain people but whose role in the pathogenesis of the syndrome is debatable.

Case history
A 45 year old woman presented with chronic right iliac fossa pain. She underwent laparotomy, during which an appendix that gave normal histological results was removed. Her pain returned in the lower abdomen three months later. A D/C, laparoscopy, and, subsequently, a hysterectomy were performed. However, pain persisted, and she volunteered that it was sometimes worse after fatty foods. Ultrasonography showed multiple gall stones and a cholecystectomy was performed. When her pain recurred she became depressed. The irritable bowel syndrome was fully diagnosed when the history was elicited of abdominal pain eased by defecation and associated with frequent, loose stools and abdominal distension. Her characteristic pain was reproduced by air insufflation at sigmoidoscopy. Long term joint management by a gastroenterologist and psychologist has helped her to control her pain reasonably and to evolve strategies to cope with her longstanding anxiety and insecurity

Natural course and follow up

Most patients with the irritable bowel syndrome do not require or wish to be followed up by a gastroenterologist. Others will require intermittent follow up, preferably by one clinician with whom they have established a rapport and who will generally be able to contain the situation, with the aid of the occasional change in treatment.

Studies of the natural course of the syndrome show that it is a safe diagnosis to make and that up to 70% of patients are virtually free of symptoms five years after presentation. In others, however, it is a chronic relapsing disorder for which permanent cure is unlikely. Most patients learn to live with their problem and find explanation and reassurance by the clinician to be the most helpful aspect of their management.

I thank Mr Alan Jackson and the staff of the medical illustration department, Bolton General Hospital, for their help in preparing the illustrations.

- The irritable bowel syndrome is a positive diagnosis, made on the basis of characteristic symptoms and signs, usually without extensive investigation
- The most important aspect of management is explanation and reassurance, allied to detection of underlying psychological factors and careful selection of treatment options

7 Haemorrhoids

B D Hancock

Haemorrhoids and related conditions are not popular with patients or doctors and are commonly relegated for treatment to a junior member of the surgical team. This is a pity because they are common and may cause considerable distress, and with expert assessment many can be cured by outpatient measures.

Haemorrhoids (or piles) are displaced anal cushions. The cushions are normal structures that have a rich arterial supply leading directly into distensible venous spaces. They help seal the upper anal canal and contribute to continence. Constipation and straining disrupt the supporting framework of the cushions, causing them to become displaced and congested. In some patients this is aggravated by a tight internal sphincter, which leads to high intra-anal pressure during a bowel action.

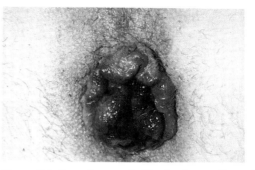

Figure 7.1 Large haemorrhoids: the dentate line, which should be halfway up the anal canal, can be clearly seen separating the prolapsed anal cushions (autonomic innervation) from the secondarily congested external plexus (somatic innervation).

Symptoms and diagnosis

Bleeding and prolapse are the cardinal symptoms of haemorrhoids. Prolapse is often the first and only symptom, and consultation is commonly deferred until bleeding starts. Bright red blood dripping into and splashed around the pan after a bowel action suggests haemorrhoids whereas darker blood mixed with the motion and with mucus strongly suggests a tumour. But history alone is unreliable for a diagnosis, and rectal examination and proctoscopy are essential before atributing the bleeding to haemorrhoids. Sigmoidoscopy is often required; this will immediately disclose ulcerative proctitis, which is the other common cause of rectal bleeding.

Bleeding is more of a problem in younger patients because the sphincter tone is higher, and haemorrhoids may occasionally cause anaemia. In older patients haemorrhoids prolapse more and may bleed only when abraded by cleaning after a bowel action. Pain, if present, suggests a thrombosis or a coexistent fissure. Irritation and soreness are understandable if piles remain prolapsed and produce some mucus or if large skin tags exist that interfere with cleaning after a bowel action. Simple pruritus ani is, however, rarely caused by haemorrhoids.

Haemorrhoids should not be diagnosed unless prolapse or bleeding is a dominant symptom, in conjunction with visibly distended or displaced anal cushions on proctoscopy. The patient should be asked to bear down to assess the degree of prolapse and to look for abnormal perineal descent, which, in its more severe form, can cause the symptoms of incomplete emptying, prolapse, or bleeding, and must not be mistaken for haemorrhoids as the treatment is different. Patients over the age of 40 and those with a family history of colorectal neoplasia who complain of rectal bleeding should undergo flexible sigmoidoscopy.

Classification of haemorrhoids

- 1st degree—bleeding only
- 2nd degree—prolapse, reduces spontaneously
- 3rd degree—prolapse, needs pushing back
- 4th degree—prolapse, permanent

This traditional classification is useful because treatment is based on symptoms rather than appearances. It is misleading, however, because prolapse often precedes bleeding by many years and some patients have acute painful prolapse lasting days but with months or years between attacks.

Investigation of rectal bleeding

Symptom	Investigation
Bright red blood:	
Seen only on paper	Inspection, rectal examination, proctoscopy and rigid sigmoidoscopy
Dripping into pan	Proctoscopy and rigid sigmoidoscopy
Mixed with motion	Proctoscopy and rigid sigmoidoscopy, flexible sigmoidoscopy
Dark red blood	Proctoscopy and flexible sigmoidoscopy, barium enema or colonoscopy optional
Anybody over 40 and those with a family history of colorectal neoplasia	**Flexible sigmoidoscopy**

Treatment

The aim is outpatient treatment, and good results can be obtained by several methods, but the best results will be obtained if the surgeon learns one or two methods really well.

Non-operative

Suppositories and ointments have little more than a placebo effect, but a high residue diet may cure many patients of early disease.

Injection and infrared coagulation

Both injection of 5% phenol in almond oil and infrared coagulation are effective for bleeding haemorrhoids with minimal prolapse. They work by tethering the cushions at the level of the anorectal junction by means of inflammation or a small controlled burn. The coagulation method is to be preferred as it is easy to use, precise, less messy than the injection method, and free from complications.

Treatment options

- *At home*
  —Suppositories
  —High residue diet
- *Outpatient*
  —Injection
  —Infrared coagulation
  —Rubber band ligation
  —Cryosurgery
- *Day case (with general anaesthesia)*
  —Dilatation and banding
  —Cryosurgery
- *Inpatient*
  —Haemorrhoidectomy

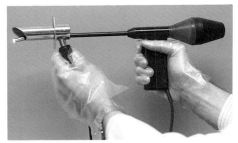

Figure 7.2 Infrared coagulator.

Simple strategy

- *Bleeding*
  —Accurate diagnosis
  —High residue diet
  —Banding or infrared coagulation optional
- *Prolapse*
  With strong sphincter
  —Dilatation and rubber band ligation under general anaesthetic as day case

  With normal sphincter
  —Rubber band ligation as an outpatient
- *Permanent prolapse*
  —Haemorrhoidectomy

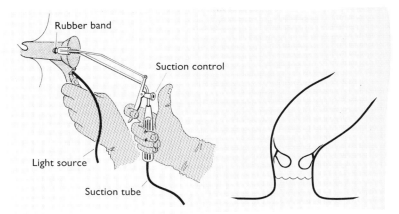

Figure 7.3 Left: suction banding instrument. The left hand controls the proctoscope while exposing the anal cushion. Suction draws some of the anal cushion into the cup and a rubber band is fired over the enclosed tissue to cause ischaemic necrosis. Right: banded haemorrhoids. Bands are placed well above the dentate line to avoid pain.

Rubber band ligation

Rubber band ligation is an alternative to haemorrhoidectomy in patients with large haemorrhoids. It works by reducing the bulk of the internal haemorrhoid. Banding requires skill in placing the bands above the dentate line to avoid severe discomfort, whereas cryosurgery may result in an unpleasant discharge for up to two weeks. The development of a suction bander has made application of the rubber bands much easier in outpatient treatment and is widely used. With this instrument it is now possible to treat more than three quarters of patients with prolapsing haemorrhoids on an outpatient basis with long term relief, provided they are prepared to suffer a little discomfort for a few days. The method may well be readily accepted when it is an alternative to haemorrhoidectomy.

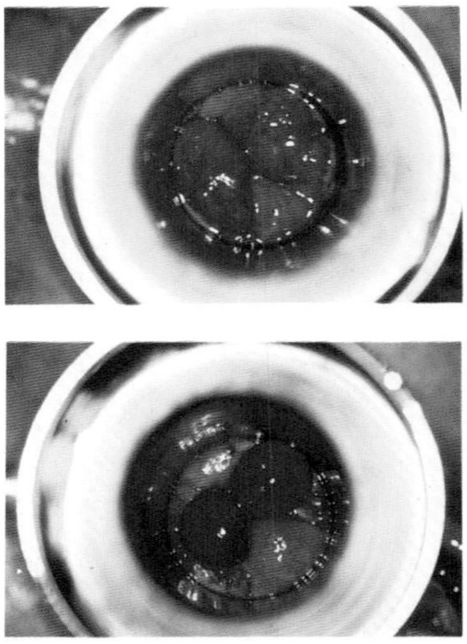

Figure 7.4 Top: the three anal cushions seen through a proctoscope before banding. Bottom: proctoscopic appearance immediately after banding. Two haemorrhoids are usually banded at the first outpatient session. The remaining one is banded three weeks later.

Anal dilatation

When the anal sphincters feel tight on rectal examination, particularly if proctoscopy causes discomfort, rubber banding as an outpatient procedure may cause too much pain. The piles can be banded more thoroughly under general anaesthetic as a day case procedure. It is usual to perform a gentle anal dilatation because anal pressure studies have shown that the internal sphincter is overactive in this sort of patient. If used with discretion and care there is no risk to the sphincter mechanism. Sequential pressure studies show that anal pressure is restored to normal and remains so for many years. With this combination of treatment excellent long term results can be expected even for large piles. Dilatation must not be done if there is any hint of weakness of the sphincter, abnormal perineal descent, or long term diarrhoea.

Haemorrhoidectomy

Haemorrhoidectomy is reserved for patients with permanent prolapse or those with large piles who want a guaranteed cure. The long term results are excellent if the operation is done skillfully, but the cost is a variable amount of postoperative pain, an inpatient stay of a few days, and two to three weeks off work.

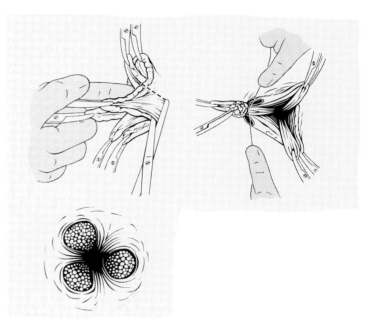

Figure 7.5 Haemorrhoidectomy. Top left: exposure of large piles before dissection. Top right: ligation after completion of dissection. Left: clover shaped perianal wound after excision of the haemorrhoid.

Care after haemorrhoid operations

Patients have traditionally stayed in hospital until the first bowel action after a haemorrhoidectomy, as the amount of pain is unpredictable. A rectal examination should be done at about one week to check there is no faecal impaction and to detect undue spasm which may precede a stenosis. Stool softeners should be provided to all patients who have had a potentially painful operation. The possibilities of day case haemorrhoidectomy and early discharge are under evaluation, and appear suitable for selected patients.

Secondary haemorrhage can occur 7–14 days after haemorrhoidectomy, banding, or cryotherapy and occasionally demands readmission for transfusion or packing. Bleeding can be controlled by inflating a Foley catheter in the rectum and strapping it to the thigh to maintain some pressure on the anorectal junction.

Care after haemorrhoidectomy

- Give adequate analgesia
- Give bulking laxative—for example, Normacol
- Patient should take frequent baths
- Perform rectal examination at about one week and again at three weeks postoperatively to check for anal stenosis and faecal impaction

---

Associated problems

Acute thrombosis

One, two, or all three piles may be affected by acute thrombosis, which may be confined to the external plexus or the whole haemorrhoid. There is usually an underlying sphincter tightness with superimposed spasm, so in the first 48 hours after thrombosis gentle anal dilatation will give great relief of pain. If this is the first attack lasting cure with dilatation can be expected, but if there is a long history of prolapse there is much to be said for an immediate haemorrhoidectomy.

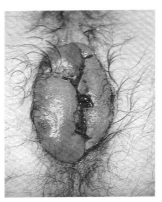

Figure 7.6 Acutely prolapsed thrombosed haemorrhoids.

Acute perianal haematoma

Acute localised thrombosis may affect the external plexus, causing a perianal haematoma. This is often caused by straining but is not associated with any internal haemorrhoids. The lesion appears as a tense blue swelling on the anal margin. Evacuation under local anaesthetic will give immediate relief, or the haematoma can be left until it discharges spontaneously.

Skin tags

Skin tags are hypertrophied redundant folds of perianal skin. They may represent the aftermath of haemorrhoids—for example, in pregnancy, though some are idiopathic and, rarely, can indicate Crohn's disease. Removal is indicated only if they cause difficulty in cleaning or irritation.

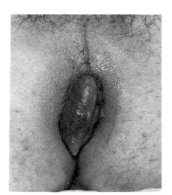

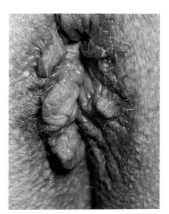

Figure 7.7 Perianal haematoma.

Figure 7.8 Anal skin tags.

8 Anal fissures and fistulas

B D Hancock

Anal fissures most commonly affect patients aged between 30 and 50. They are equally common in men and women. A fissure is a split in the lower half of the anal canal extending from the anal verge towards the dentate line. Most fissures are posterior, but anterior ones are often seen in women. The cause is not clear, but a fissure often starts after an attack of either diarrhoea or constipation. Some heal spontaneously but many become chronic, causing months of misery.

Reflex spasm of the external sphincter occurs whenever the fissure is disturbed. There is also a background tightness of the internal sphincter, which may well be the primary fault because correction of this abnormality almost always cures the fissure. The base of the fissure has somatic innervation, so pain can become intense after a bowel action and last as a dull pain for many hours. A chronic intersphincteric abscess can cause a similar sort of pain, but pain severe enough to warrant emergency admission to hospital must be assumed to be caused by a high anorectal abscess.

Diagnosis

Unless there is intense spasm, the lower end of a fissure will come into view with the patient in the left lateral position as the perianal skin is gently retracted. After a time the skin at the base of the fissure becomes oedematous and hypertrophied, forming a sentinel pile. A limited rectal examination to assess the degree of spasm is useful because this is an important guide to treatment, but it is often impossible because of pain.

Symptoms of anal fissure

- Anal pain during and after bowel action
- Minor bleeding
- Irritation
- Constipation

Treatment

If there is little spasm, correction of constipation with a bulking agent aided by a topical anaesthetic is usually sufficient. Relapse is quite common. Minor surgery should be offered to those with servere pain and spasm from the outset or if symptoms have been present for one month.

Gentle dilatation of the anus and lateral subcutaneous sphincterotomy are both effective for correction of internal sphincter tightness as day case procedures. Both methods work by reducing resting anal pressure to normal. The sentinel pile should be excised if present. In controlled trials anal dilatation has been shown to be slightly inferior to lateral subcutaneous sphincterotomy with respect to recurrence rate and the incidence of minor complications such as lack of control of flatus. Permanent cure can be expected, but a long term high fibre diet is advisable.

Topical 0.2% GTN cream applied to the anus is proving to be an effective alternative to both sphincterotomy and dilatation. Headaches can be a disabling side effect, but many patients tolerate the treatment because their fissure and associated pain resolves obviating the need for a surgical procedure.

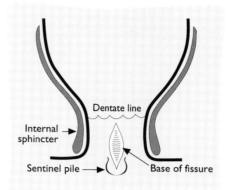

Figure 8.1 Anal fissure—a vertical split in the squamous lined lower half of the anal canal.

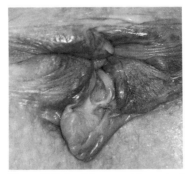

Figure 8.2 Anal fissure with sentinel pile.

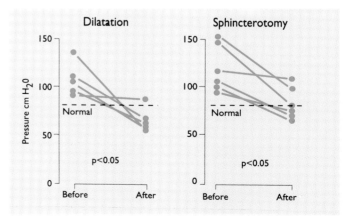

Figure 8.3 Anal pressures before and after procedures for fissure. The high pretreatment values may induce local ischaemia sufficient to prevent spontaneous healing.

Anorectal abscesses and fistulas

An abscess and a fistula are respectively the acute and chronic sequelae of an infected anal gland. About 10 glands drain into the anal canal at the level of the dentate line. Some penetrate the internal sphincter to reach the intersphincteric space.

The common perianal abscess comprises downward spread between the internal and external sphincter. In the 5% of patients in whom infection spreads upwards between the sphincters increasing pain is prominent. There are no external signs and a rectal examination may be painful but is diagnostic.

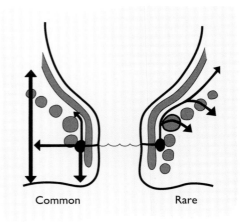

Figure 8.4 Anal canal showing spread of infection from gland.

By the time symptoms have been present for 24 hours incision and drainage are required. Antibiotics rarely abort the infection. A fulminating infection may occur in immunocompromised and diabetic patients and requires broad spectrum antibiotics and generous drainage.

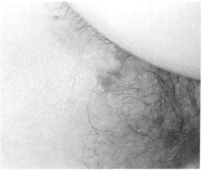

Figure 8.5 Perianal abscesses.

In general, anorectal abscesses do not require wide incision, nor does the cavity need to be packed. Recurrence occurs in up to 25% of patients because there is still a tiny communication between the infected anal gland and the anal canal (a fistula). The opening is often minute. It is unwise to look for it when the abscess is drained because it is easy to make a false passage with a probe. If the abscess is recurrent, and especially if *Escherichia coli* is grown from the pus, the chance of a fistula is high, so the patient should be examined in the operating room one week after drainage to find the fistula and lay it open to prevent further recurrence.

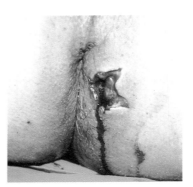

Figure 8.6 Drained perianal abscess.

Anal fistulas

Many fistulas start as an abscess; others develop insidiously. A few are caused by Crohn's disease, which is usually active in the colon or, occasionally, just in the terminal ileum. Rarely, fistulas are caused by trauma, tuberculosis, or a neglected carcinoma. The symptoms are persistent or recurrent discharge or abscess in the perianal region. In chronic intersphincteric abscesses, which are uncommon, the discharge is from the anus itself.

Most fistulas have a fairly straight track between an external opening close to the anus and an internal opening in the anal canal at the level of the anal valves. The internal opening in about one third of fistulas is tiny or stenosed, but if it is not found and excised along with the chronically infected intersphincteric gland recurrence is common. In practice, careful probing with lachrymal probes, following granulation tissue or using dilute methylene blue, will suffice. Recent studies have shown that magnetic resonance imaging reliably shows the tracks in problematic cases. The track is simply laid open, dividing the lower portion of the sphincters. The wound edges are trimmed to leave a shallow, pear shaped wound.

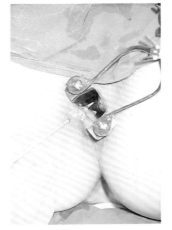

Figure 8.7 Anal fistula.

About 5% of fistulas have complex branching tracts passing high up through the sphincter complex, and initial attempts at surgery often fail because of inadequate exploration of tracks for fear of producing incontinence.

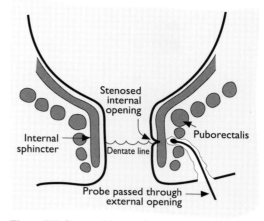

Figure 8.8 Stenosed internal opening.

Features of a complex fistula
- Recurrent trouble after surgery
- Multiple external openings
- Induration felt above puborectalis
- Probe from external opening passes vertically upwards instead of towards the mid-anal canal

---

The puborectalis sling, which maintains a right angle at the anorectal junction, is the most important component of anal continence. Provided it is intact there will be no major loss of continence. Occasionally a fistula passes over or through the puborectalis, and if it were laid open in one stage continence would certainly be at risk. This is an unacceptable price to pay for cure of a fistula.

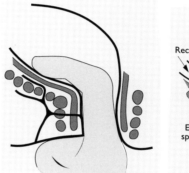

Figure 8.9 Palpation of high tracts on rectal examination.

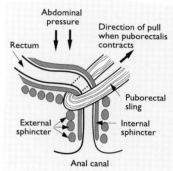

Figure 8.10 Puborectalis sling around the anorectal junction.

Many ingenious methods have been devised to preserve the external sphincter complex when the puborectalis is affected, but unfortunately they all seem to have an appreciable associated recurrence rate. The fistula can be cured, however, provided the tracks are fully explored and laid open in stages.

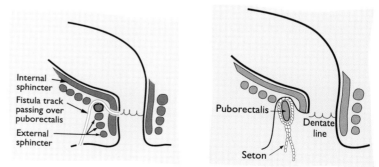

Figure 8.11 Laying open the fistula track. A seton of silk suture is passed through the suprasphincteric track and tied around the fistula track. The lower part of the fistula track has been laid open. The suture is replaced and tightened at intervals of a few weeks until it cuts out. The puborectalis muscle does not spring apart as it would if divided in one stage.

After care

The simple fistula wound requires nothing more than regular baths and a gauze swab moistened with an antiseptic solution applied to the wound once a day. The care of a complex fistula wound is the responsibility of the surgeon and should not be delegated to the district nurse. The deep anal wound necessary to lay open a high track must not be allowed to close down too soon on the outside. This demands proper shaping of the wound. A dressing can be done in the operating room after five or six days. Thereafter the surgeon should check with his or her finger at the daily dressing that no deep cavities or pockets are reforming. A dressing is simply laid in. This may need a longer period in hospital but is a small price to pay for cure of a troublesome fistula.

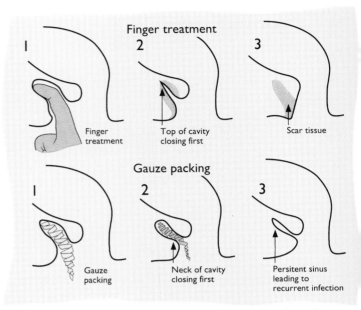

Figure 8.12 Ribbon gauze packing may be harmful by keeping a deep wound open. Gentle exploration with the finger keeps the cavity open to encourage healing from the bottom.

Crohn's perianal fistulas

Crohn's perianal fistula presents a special problem. It has a distinctive appearance, with more oedema and opening, and surprisingly little discomfort. If there is active Crohn's disease in the colon or rectum a surgical wound in the anus may never heal. Provided the intestinal Crohn's disease can be brought under control by steroids, sulphasalazine, or appropriate surgery, the fistula can be treated conventionally. If disease continues in the colon, troublesome anal sepsis or fistula may tip the balance in favour of an early panproctocolectomy.

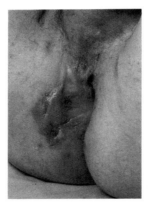

Figure 8.13 Perianal fistula in Crohn's disease.

9   Pilonidal sinus

D J Jones

Pilonidal disease is a common affliction of young adults that causes considerable suffering, inconvenience, and time lost from work. Treatment varies greatly and is often less than satisfactory. The rate of recurrence after surgery is purported to be as high as 50%.

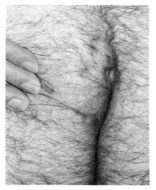

Figure 9.1 Pilonidal sinus.

What is a pilonidal sinus?

A pilonidal sinus consists of a characteristic midline opening or series of openings in the natal cleft about 5 cm from the anus. The skin enters the sinus, giving the opening a smooth edge. This primary track leads into a subcutaneous cavity which contains granulation tissue and usually a nest of hairs, which may be seen projecting through the skin opening. Many patients have secondary lateral openings 2–5 cm from the midline pit. The skin opening and superficial portion of the track are lined with squamous cell epithelium, but the deep cavity and its extensions are not.

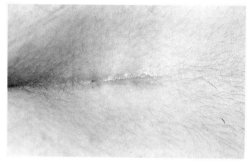

Figure 9.2 Non-infected pilonidal sinus.

Pathogenesis

Pilonidal sinuses are now widely accepted as being acquired abnormalities, although theories of a congenital origin, from postcoccygeal cells or vestigial scent glands, were once popular. Sinuses to the neural canal and dura are rare; they usually present in childhood and are in the lumbar rather than the sacral region.

Pilonidal disease starts at the onset of puberty, when sex hormones start acting on pilosebaceous glands in the natal cleft. A hair follicle becomes distended with keratin and subsequently infected, leading to a folliculitis and an abscess which extends down into the subcutaneous fat. Tracks spread out of the cavity in the direction of the neighbouring hair growth, which is towards the patient's head in over 90% of cases. A small proportion have tracks which pass caudally, and these pilonidal sinuses tend to be closer to the anus. Hairs are drilled or sucked into the cavity owing to friction with movement of the buttocks. Barbs on the hairs prevent their expulsion, so that they become trapped, provoking a foreign body type reaction and infection.

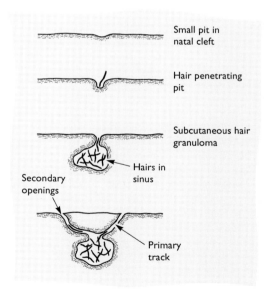

Small pit in natal cleft

Hair penetrating pit

Subcutaneous hair granuloma

Hairs in sinus

Secondary openings

Primary track

Figure 9.3 Mechanism of pathogenesis of a pilonidal sinus.

Clinical features

Pilonidal sinuses present from the age of puberty to about 40 years of age, but rarely in older people. Three quarters of patients are men, predominantly in their 20s. About 1% of men in the age group at risk develop a pilonidal sinus. Affected women tend to be younger, which is consistent with their earlier onset of puberty. Patients are usually, but not invariably, dark and hairy, and are often obese. Pilonidal sinuses are less common among Africans and Asians owing to different hair characteristics and growth patterns.

Half of the affected patients present as emergencies with an acute pilonidal abscess; the remainder have fluctuating discomfort and chronic infection with a foul smelling discharge. Examination reveals the characteristic opening in the natal cleft, through which a tuft of hair may be seen emerging.

Treatment

Many different treatments have been advocated with conflicting enthusiasm, suggesting that none is perfect. Some patients can be treated on an outpatient or day case basis whereas others require periods in hospital. A balance has to be struck between minimising inpatient treatment without compromising lasting healing. The best results will be obtained if the surgeon learns one or two methods really well.

Curettage
If the sinus is small and not infected hairs can be removed by using forceps or small bristle brushes and the surrounding skin is shaved weekly. In the absence of a persisting foreign body reaction to the hair, healing may occur.

Excision
Excision of pits—Midline pits and lateral openings can be excised with a small area (less than 0·5 cm) of surrounding skin under local anaesthesia and the cavity curetted to remove the hair granuloma. The sinus requires frequent changes of dressings and weekly brushing with a small bristle brush. Healing occurs in about six weeks.

Laying open—If the acquired theory of aetiology is accepted it is not necessary to perform an excision down to the presacral fascia. Laying the sinus open to permit adequate drainage allows healing by secondary intention. Frequent changes of dressings and close supervision are necessary to prevent pocketing. Regular rubbing with a finger avoids premature closure or bridging of the skin edges over an incompletely healed cavity; these tend to occur as healing nears completion, when attention to the wound is waning.

Excision with primary suture—The pilonidal sinus is excised and the wound sutured under general anaesthesia by using deep tension sutures tied over a gauze dressing. This approximates the skin edges and occludes the dead space where blood and serum could collect and become infected. Broad spectrum prophylactic antibiotics are prescribed to minimise the risks of infection. Many doctors advocate a low residue diet to minimise defecation and faecal contamination of the wound in the early postoperative period. Primary closure requires a longer period in hospital with up to one week of bed rest. Patients who accept this are rewarded with early complete healing after two weeks. This method is particularly suited to patients who find it difficult to accept an open wound. If the wound becomes infected it is reopened and allowed to heal by secondary intention. However, delayed healing may occur if the wound becomes infected but is not laid open. Many patients undoubtedly benefit from primary closure, but the proportions healed at two months are similar for open and closed methods of treatment.

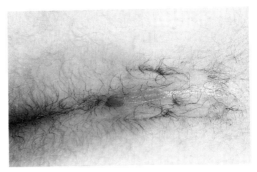
Figure 9.4 Pilonidal sinus with discharge.

> Meticulous hygiene and shaving are important for all forms of treatment. Shaving may be stopped once the wound has healed

Management of open granulating wounds
- Adequate drainage combined with the prevention of pocketing and bridging are more important than the type of dressing used
- Tight packing is contraindicated as it prevents wound drainage and causes discomfort

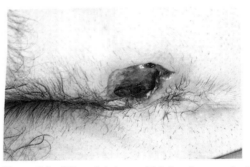
Figure 9.5 Pilonodal sinus which has been excised and left open to heal by secondary intention. Further shaving around the cavity is needed.

Principal surgical options
Non-infected sinus
  Excision and primary closure
  Excision and laying open
Infected sinus or abscess
  Drainage and excision
  Healing by secondary intention

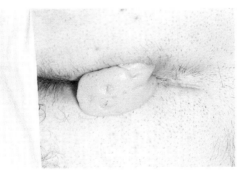
Figure 9.6 Laid open pilonodal sinus with a dressing of Silastic foam.

Excision with primary suture and flattening of the natal cleft—
Techniques that flatten the natal cleft help to diminish the accumulation of hair and reduce friction with movement. The sinus is excised asymmetrically, with one flap being undermined and overlapped over the opposite flap. Alternatively a myocutaneous flap or Z-plasty flap can be used to close the wound. These techniques are more demanding and require a period in hospital. If the operation is unsuccessful patients endure a more prolonged period of healing owing to the size and complexity of the wound.

Causes of recurrence

Early recurrence is usually the result of the persistence of tracks lined with granulation tissue in an incompletely healed wound. Late recurrence is caused by repeated infection of hair follicles. Procedures that leave a midline scar are most susceptible to further hair penetration. Healing by secondary intention leaves a flat, broad, hairless scar which reduces buttock friction and is less susceptible to penetration by hair.

Pilonidal abscess

A pilonidal abscess is incised, drained, and curetted free of hairs and granulation tissue. Complete healing occurs within one month, but almost a third of patients develop a pilonidal sinus and require further treatment.

Recurrence is reduced if sinus pits are recognised and excised at the time of primary drainage, although these may be dificult to recognise in the presence of infection and oedema. The pit is more easily distinguished and excised a week after primary drainage, when the oedema has resolved. This reduces the patient's chance of developing a chronic sinus and avoids readmission.

Comparison of primary closure and laying open

Primary closure	*Laying open*
Quicker healing	Slower healing
Success depends on the surgeon	Effective in most hands
Early return to work	Open wound may delay return to work
Failure delays healing	
Longer period in hospital	Shorter period in hospital
Minimal wound care	Active wound care with frequent wound dressings

The proportions healed at two months are similar for both forms of treatment

---

Causes of recurrence
- Neglect of wound care
- Persisting poorly drained tracks
- Recurrent infection of hair follicles
- Midline scars

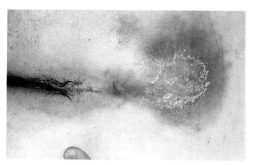

Figure 9.7 Pilonidal abscess.

10 Pruritus ani

N M Craven, D J Jones

Pruritus ani is a common and frustrating symptom, with sensations of itch, burning, or even pain around the anus. One to five per cent of the population are affected; it is more common in men than women (4:1), and usually presents in the fourth, fifth, and sixth decades. Although the aetiology of the condition is not fully understood, and in any one patient may be the result of the interaction of several factors, most patients can be helped by education and relatively straightforward therapeutic measures.

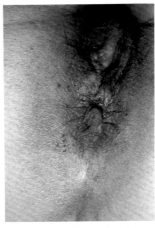

Figure 10.1 Mild perianal excoriation.

Aetiology

About 50% of patients with pruritus ani do not have a discernible cause for their condition. Several factors probably play a part in such patients: faecal contamination from poor personal hygiene, moisture from sweat, exudate or anal leakage, friction, and other trauma to the skin. Dietary factors have been implicated (see box) and psychogenic factors often appear to play a role.

Dietary factors implicated in pruritus ani	
Coffee	Tea
Cola	Chocolate
Alcohol	Spices
Milk	Pork
Tomatoes	Corn
Nuts	Citrus fruits
Drugs	
colchicine	
quinidine	
antibiotics	
laxatives	
mineral oil	

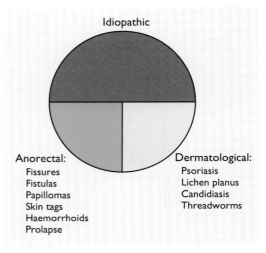

Figure 10.2 Aetiology of pruritus ani.

A number of patients have an easily recognisable condition such as anal fissures, anal fistulae, papillomas, skin tags, prolapsing haemorrhoids, or rectal prolapse. Any condition that hampers efficient wiping of the anus may allow small particles of faeces to accumulate on the perianal skin and act as an irritant.

Pruritus ani may be a manifestation of a dermatological disorder such as psoriasis, seborrhoeic dermatitis, allergic contact dermatitis to topically applied medications, lichen sclerosus, lichen planus, Bowen's disease, or Paget's disease. Infections and infestations such as tinea cruris, candidiasis, erythrasma, threadworms, pediculosis pubis, and scabies are easily treatable but also easily overlooked causes of pruritus ani.

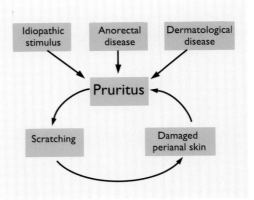

Figure 10.3 Evolution of pruritus ani.

Clinical features

Patients develop a slight itch in the perianal skin, which may progress to severe pruritus over the entire perineum. Symptoms are usually worse at night, when they may be the sole focus of attention. The condition is often worse during the summer, when sweating is greatest. The patient eases the itch by scratching the perineum, thereby producing short lived relief. Continued scratching causes damaging excoriations which may bleed. A vicious circle of itching and scratching develops which is difficult to break.

Examination of the perianal area may, in some cases, show a normal appearance, but will usually reveal changes resulting from scratching or rubbing. In the acute stage the skin may show erythema, oedema, maceration, excoriations, and in extreme cases a weeping eroded dermatitis. Chronic rubbing leads to lichenification with exaggeration of the skin folds and creases around the anus.

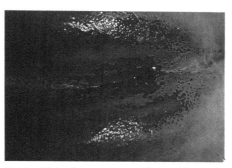

Figure 10.4 Severe contact dermatitis caused by topical antiseptics which had been used to treat pruritus ani.

Management

Important aetiological factors may be ascertained from the history by paying particular attention to dietary factors, topical medications applied, personal hygiene measures, bowel habit, and other gastrointestinal or dermatological symptoms.

A thorough anorectal examination is performed to identify potentially correctable anatomical problems. Lesions such as haemorrhoids and tags should be treated surgically, with the aim of achieving a smooth anus that can be wiped easily, and where faeces cannot accumulate. The patient should be examined for evidence of primary dermatological disorders, and in this respect examination of skin and mucous membranes in other areas is desirable.

Threadworms appear as thin white threads about 6 mm in length and may be seen around the anal orifice. They can also be identified in the effluent of a diagnostic saline enema. If threadworms are discovered, patients and their families are treated with a course of mebendazole and strict measures of hygiene adopted to prevent reinfection. Pediculosis pubis is treated with topical malathion, and scabies with topical malathion or permethrin cream. Close contacts should be treated simultaneously.

If the reddened skin has a clearly demarcated margin, the possibility of fungal infection should be investigated by microscopic examination and culture of skin scrapings. If confirmed, treatment is with a topical antifungal agent. Candida infection should be treated using a combination of oral and topical nystatin.

Referral for patch testing is indicated if there is any suspicion that a patient has become sensitised to topical medicaments or toiletries. A skin biopsy may help with the diagnosis in selected cases, particularly if changes in the perianal skin are asymmetrical.

Many patients will not have an identifiable lesion to treat, and many who undergo surgery for potentially implicated anorectal conditions continue to have symptoms. These patients should receive guidance on general measures to improve care of the perianal skin.

All currently used topical preparations should be discontinued. After defecation, the patient should clean the perianal skin by gentle washing in warm water or by using moistened cotton wool. The skin should be patted dry with cotton gauze or toilet tissue and rubbing should be

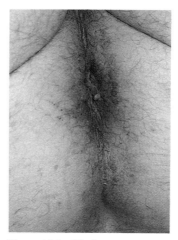

Figure 10.5 Discharge associated with papillomas is a common cause of pruritus ani. Treatment of the papillomas relieves itching.

> **Management of pruritus ani**
> - Identify and treat secondary causes
> - Give advice about personal hygiene
> - Maintain the patient's confidence
> - Avoid frequent unproductive clinic visits

avoided. If the perianal skin is acutely inflamed, 0·25% silver nitrate solution has a useful astringent effect when applied to the affected area and allowed to dry. This should be followed by the application of 1% hydrocortisone cream, although in some cases a short course of moderately potent topical steroid such as 0·05% clobetasone butyrate (Eumovate cream) may be required. Prolonged use of fluorinated steroids should be avoided because they may readily produce atrophy in this occluded area. Zinc paste with 2% phenol has a helpful protective and antipruritic effect and may benefit patients prone to problems with leakage. It should be applied before and after defecation, and again at night. Other local applications such as calamine lotion and carbolic lotion may soothe the perineum, break the vicious circle of itching and scratching, and allow the damaged skin to heal. Topical anaesthetics and antihistamines should be avoided as they can induce allergic contact dermatitis. Some authorities recommend the use of a small cotton pledget applied to the anus to keep the area dry. This can be dusted with Zeasorb powder or cornflour to prevent sticking to the skin.

The patient should be advised to avoid tight or restrictive clothing. A bulking agent may help to produce a soft bulky stool. Exclusion of dietary factors thought to predispose to pruritus ani should be maintained for two weeks before the foods are reintroduced in small quantities, increasing up to the level of tolerance. Sedative antihistamines may be helpful at night, and soft cotton gloves worn overnight will reduce damage from scratching during sleep.

Providing the patient with simple printed guidelines can improve the chances of success (see box). Strict adherence to such advice undoubtedly helps, and the regimen may be relaxed as symptoms ease. Some patients neverless continue to suffer, and may become obsessional about their bowel habit and perineum.

Guidelines for patients with pruritus ani

- Keep the anal area clean by gentle washing and drying after defecation
- Soap can irritate the skin, and perfumes in soap can cause allergies which may make your symptoms worse
- Use only specifically prescribed creams and ointments, as some preparations may be allergenic
- Avoid impervious underwear such as acrylic and nylon garments which trap sweat
- Maintain a regular bowel habit
- Some foods and drinks are thought to cause pruritus ani in some patients. The following are most frequently suspected, especially if taken in large quantities: coffee, tea, cola, beer, chocolate, tomatoes (and ketchup), spicy foods. Try cutting each one out of the diet for two weeks, then slowly reintroducing them in increasing quantities. In this way, you can find out how much your body can tolerate without producing symptoms
- Wear cotton gloves at night to reduce the damage from scratching during sleep. Your doctor may be able to give you an antihistamine to take at night if symptoms disturb sleep

---

For patients with intractable pruritus ani resistant to such measures, various other approaches have been advocated including injection of alcohol or phenol into the perianal skin to destroy the subcutaneous nerves, and cryotherapy. The results are variable, but lasting benefit is obtained in some cases.

Patients sometimes tend to make repeated visits to outpatient clinics with little improvement, seeing a different doctor at each visit. There is a danger that they will become disillusioned. An honest approach is best, warning the patient that a precise cause for their condition may not be found but that by paying attention to personal hygiene their symptoms can be minimised. In chronic cases a dermatological opinion is valuable to be sure that a skin condition such as psoriasis is not being missed.

11 Rectal Prolapse

J H Hobbiss, D J Jones

Rectal prolapse is an uncommon condition that usually occurs at the extreme ends of life, particularly in elderly women and infants. There are three degrees of rectal prolapse: complete or full thickness, incomplete or mucosal, and concealed.

Complete rectal prolapse—This occurs when there is intussusception of the lower rectum through the anus. The prolapse consists of two full thickness layers of rectal wall.

Incomplete rectal prolapse—This occurs when only the mucosa protrudes through the anal canal.

Concealed rectal prolapse—This occurs when there is an internal intussusception of the lower rectum with straining. The mucosa of the lower rectum does not prolapse through the anal canal, but may be trapped against the closed canal causing ulceration. This is known as the solitary rectal ulcer syndrome.

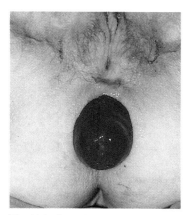

Fig 11.1 Complete rectal prolapse.

Aetiology

Rectal prolapse occurs when there is a rise in the intra-abdominal pressure, commonly during straining at stool, which overcomes the muscular and ligamentous support structures that normally fix the rectum into the pelvis. Predisposing and associated factors include those in the box.

Although rectal prolapse is six times more common in women than in men, it is not associated with childbirth or parity.

In infancy, when there is immaturity of the anatomical structures that support the rectum in the pelvic region, rectal prolapse usually occurs with constipation and straining at stool. Infants with cystic fibrosis are particularly prone to rectal prolapse, which may occasionally be the first clinical manifestation of this condition.

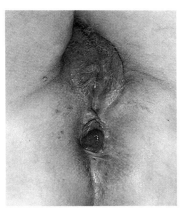

Fig 11.2 Incomplete rectal prolapse.

Predisposing factors

Constipation

Excessive straining at stool

Female sex

Deep pouch of Douglas

Redundant sigmoid colon

Decreased anal sphincter tone

Reduced pelvic floor support

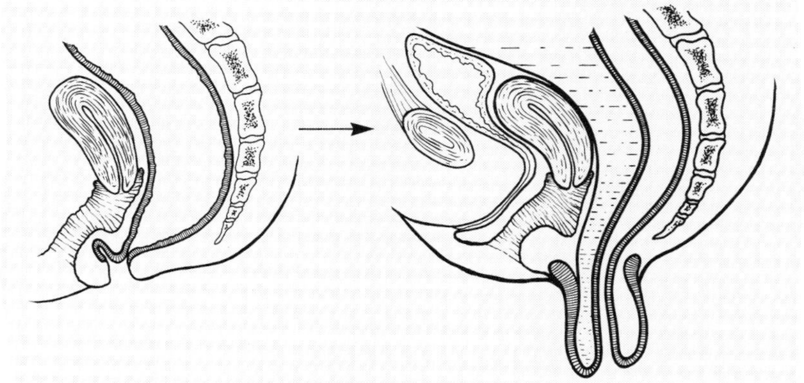

Fig 11.3 Probable evolution of rectal prolapse. Internal prolapse of rectum into upper anal canal (left) ultimately becomes a complete prolapse of the rectum through the anus (right).

Clinical features

Adults

Most adults present with a prolapse resulting from defecation which reduces spontaneously or with manual assistance. In more advanced cases, prolapse may occur with exercise or coughing and only reduces if the patient lies down. Occasionally, the prolapse is irreducible and urgent hospital admission is required. Prolapse causes perianal discomfort, mucus discharge, bleeding, and perianal excoriation. Three quarters of patients with rectal prolapse also have faecal incontinence.

Children

Prolapse is usually noticed by the parent after the infant has defecated; initially it causes a great deal of anxiety. It is usually easily reduced.

Examination

The prolapse is not usually visible when the patient is first examined. It may sometimes be demonstrated by asking the patient to strain while in the left lateral position. Initially abnormal perineal descent and a patulous anus may be noted and the prolapse may take several minutes to emerge through the anus. Sometimes the patient has to sit on the lavatory seat and strain. Complete rectal prolapse is recognised by its concentric mucosal rings. In mucosal prolapse the protruding mucosa may not be circumferential and has radial folds.

The anus is lax on digital examination with reduced voluntary contraction. Proctitis secondary to the trauma of prolapse is a common finding on sigmoidoscopy. The differential diagnosis of rectal prolapse includes prolapsing haemorrhoids, prolapsing rectal polyps, or rarely malignant tumours and perianal warts. These are readily distinguished on rectal examination and proctoscopy.

Treatment

Adults

Patients who have only occasional episodes of prolapse are best treated with bulk laxatives to produce defecation without straining. Patients in whom the prolapse occurs sufficiently frequently for it to be a nuisance and those in whom it is difficult to reduce should be referred for surgical treatment. Rarely a patient presents with a gangrenous prolapse requiring urgent surgical treatment. The faecal incontinence often associated with rectal prolapse may improve after surgery. The incontinence problem is, therefore, usually reassessed after prolapse repair, rather than attempting to deal with the two problems together.

Children

In children prolapse usually resolves with dietary advice and toilet training. This may require admission to hospital but surgery is rarely required.

Surgery

A large number of operations have been described and advocated with varying degrees of enthusiasm, suggesting that none is perfect. Surgical procedures for rectal prolapse may be performed by either the perineal or the abdominal approach. The perineal operations are less invasive and this can be an important advantage, especially in the elderly, although recurrence rates may be higher.

Clinical features

Symptoms
- Prolapse initially related to defecation
- Mucus discharge
- Bleeding
- Incontinence

Signs
- Patulous anus
- Perianal excoriation
- Reduced anal tone
- Increased perineal descent on straining
- Visible prolapse in advanced cases

Other conditions that may cause prolapse through the anus
- Large haemorrhoids
- Prolapsing rectal tumour
- Anal warts
- Abnormal perineal descent
- Anal polyps

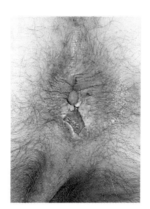

Fig 11.4 Prolapsing anal polyp.

Operations for rectal prolapse

Incomplete prolapse
—Injection sclerotherapy
—Haemorrhoidectomy

Complete prolapse
Perineal operation:
—Thiersch suture
—Delorme operation
—Perineal rectopexy

Abdominal operation:
—Abdominal rectopexy
—Anterior resection rectopexy

Perineal operations

Delorme procedure—In the Delorme procedure, the mucosa is stripped off the prolapsed rectum and the underlying muscle is plicated with multiple sutures. This effectively controls the prolapse in the short term, but recurrence may occur with time. Recurrences can be treated with a further Delorme procedure if necessary. The Delorme procedure has the major advantage of being a relatively painless operation and is well tolerated in elderly patients. A modification of the Delorme procedure can be used in mucosal prolapse whereby the prolapsing mucosa is dissected off the underlying rectal wall in the submucosal plane and the proximal mucosal end is sutured to the mucosa just above the anorectal junction.

Perineal resection—Perineal rectosigmoidectomy, together with a coloanal anastomosis, may be performed when there is a very large prolapse in a patient who is unfit for abdominal surgery. This is an effective operation, but there is a tendency for recurrence with time, although usually to a much lesser degree.

Perianal suture—The insertion of an encircling (Thiersch) suture was once popular. It has now largely been abandoned because of poor functional results.

Abdominal operations

Abdominal rectopexy—This was once the most popular operation for those patients fit enough for laparotomy. The rectum is mobilised and attached to the sacrum by sutures or synthetic material, usually polypropylene mesh (Ripstein) or Ivalon sponge (Wells). This is effective in controlling the prolapse in both the short and the long term. The main disadvantage of this procedure is that it tends to increase the constipation and straining which these patients often already have. The operation may now be performed by laparoscopy.

Anterior resection rectopexy—Resection of the sigmoid loop and upper rectum gives superior results, especially in patients with defective colonic transit. It is not necessary to use prosthetic materials and postoperative constipation and straining are largely avoided. The main disadvantage of this operation is that resection and anastomosis increase the potential for complications.

Solitary rectal ulcer syndrome

Solitary rectal ulcer syndrome is a chronic inflammation, sometimes amounting to frank ulceration on the anterior wall of the lower rectum. Biopsies demonstrate a characteristic pattern of fibromuscular obliteration of the lamina propria. Using defecating proctography the aetiology of this inflammation has been demonstrated as concealed anterior mucosal prolapse during straining at stool; this is then traumatised against the top end of the anal canal.

Solitary rectal ulcer syndrome is equally common in men and women, with a peak incidence in the fourth decade. The clinical features are of bleeding and mucus discharge in a patient who has difficulty with defecation. It can be distinguished from ulcerative proctitis by its localisation to the anterior wall of the lower rectum and by its characteristic histological appearance.

Management

Constipation is treated and patients are advised to avoid excessive straining at stool. Many topical treatments, including steroid enemas, have been used, but none significantly affects

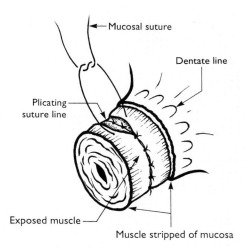

Fig 11.5 Delorme procedure: the prolapsing mucosa is dissected off the underlying muscle. The muscle is plicated with sutures and the mucosa anastomosed.

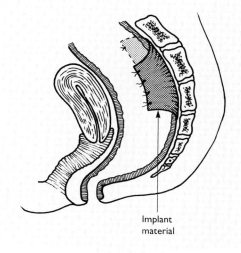

Fig 11.6 Rectopexy.

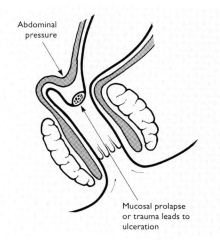

Fig 11.7 Possible aetiology of solitary rectal ulcer.

the course of the disease. Symptoms tend to be intermittent and a nuisance. The underlying difficulty in defecation may be more disabling. Surgery is indicated only rarely in the most severe cases, in which excisional rectopexy may be necessary.

Proctalgia fugax

Proctalgia fugax is characterised by attacks of severe pain in the rectum, perineum, or urethra. It occurs suddenly, often at night, waking the patient up. The pain rises to a crescendo over a few minutes and then subsides. It is often familial and commonly affects healthy men. It is probably caused by spasms in the muscles of the perineal floor. It is not related to any disorder of defecation.

Treatment, after exclusion of other organic disease, is centred on explanation of the symptoms and reassurance of the patient that there is no serious underlying pathology. Analgesics or glyceryl trinitrate may be tried if necessary, but the pain has usually passed off before they become effective. In severe cases the patient may be taught to insert a gloved finger into the anal canal to stretch the puborectalis muscle, in much the same way as a person forcibly extends the calf muscles in an attack of cramp.

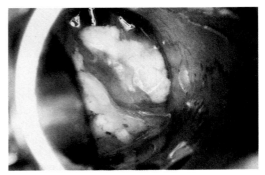

Fig 11.8 White indurated base of a solitary rectal ulcer viewed through a proctoscope.

Treatment of proctalgia fugax

- Explanation and reassurance
- Analgesics
- Antispasmodics
- Glyceryl trinitrate
- Puborectalis stretch

---

12 Faecal Incontinence

E S Kiff

The distress associated with faecal incontinence needs no imagination. The frequency with which it is today seen in colorectal clinics implies that in times gone by those afflicted suffered in silence rather than face the embarrassment of discussing the problem with a doctor. Happily, today more is known abut the condition so that in many instances the condition can be totally alleviated or substantially improved.

Aetiology

Faecal incontinence can be defined as the uncontrolled passage of stool through the rectum from either a lack of awareness of the need to defecate (cerebral or peripheral) or an inability to get to a lavatory in time, which may be the result of the rapid transit through the bowel (for example, diarrhoea), poor rectal capacity (for example, chronic proctitis), or poor anal sphincter activity (for example, as a result of rectal prolapse or after obstetric sphincter injury or fistula surgery). In many such cases treatment of the underlying condition cures the incontinence.

Faecal incontinence in elderly people is commonly associated with an impacted rectum and alleviated in most by disimpaction. It has been suggested that both the faecal impaction and incontinence are the result of a local sensory deficit.

There remains a large group of patients, who are otherwise fit and well, whose faecal incontinence is, at first sight, of unknown aetiology. Such patients are grossly incapacitated by their symptoms and yet many can be cured. There is accumulating evidence that many of these patients have suffered damage to the pudendal nerves.

The key to success here is to keep the stool as formed as possible and to initiate defecation with suppositories on a regular basis.

This approach can also be successful in the management of patients with multiple sclerosis, whose pelvic floor and sphincter mechanism is neither good enough to allow easy defecation of a solid stool nor strong enough to prevent incontinence of a loose stool.

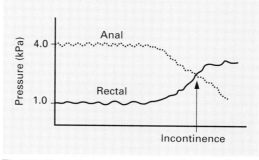

Fig 12.1 Faecal incontinence occurs when rectal pressure exceeds anal pressure.

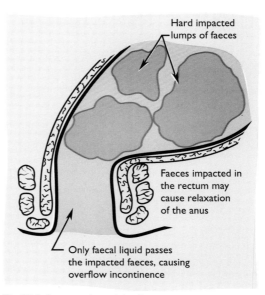

Hard impacted lumps of faeces

Faeces impacted in the rectum may cause relaxation of the anus

Only faecal liquid passes the impacted faeces, causing overflow incontinence

Fig 12.2 Impacted stool in the rectum.

Investigation

Despite it being virtually a daily occurrence for us all, people do not like to talk about defecation. Consequently, patients with faecal incontinence are embarrassed about it and tend to suffer their symptoms for many years. It is important to ask the right questions. One should enquire about the nature of the call to stool—it is often altered or lost in neuropathic incontinence. Urgency of defecation, with often only a few minutes warning, in the presence of a solid stool suggests voluntary muscle weakness. Difficulty in wiping the anus indicates a lax sphincter or prolapse. Leakage between defecatory episodes—initially for flatus but eventually for solid stool—indicates low sphincter tone at rest (RT) and usually internal sphincter deficiency. Stress incontinence on coughing, bending, or walking suggests voluntary muscle weakness.

Factors to ask about
- Call to stool
- Urgency
- Consistency of stools
- Difficulty wiping
- Leakage
- Urinary incontinence
- Obstetric history
- Anal surgery

Most patients with idiopathic faecal incontinence are women and many have had one or more difficult deliveries. In most cases there is evidence of pudendal neuropathy. About half of these patients will also have a history of urinary incontinence. It is probable that the aetiology is the same because many women with urinary incontinence alone have evidence of subclinical damage to the innervation of the anal sphincters. A history of anal surgery, particularly anal dilatation, which can damage the internal sphincter, and fistula surgery may be significant.

Observation and digital examination

Together with the history, anal examination with the eye and the index finger will frequently lead to a diagnosis.

Perianal soiling should alert the doctor to the possibility of faecal incontinence. Gaping of the anus at rest or on perianal traction means low sphincter tone at rest and therefore poor internal sphincter function. Descent of the anal verge below the level of the ischial tuberosities suggests muscle weakness of the pelvic floor. Straining down by the patient may accentuate this or may reveal a rectal prolapse. Scars may mean underlying muscle division.

Digital examination is obligatory. If inserting the gloved finger is easy, the sphincter tone at rest is low and therefore the internal sphincter is poor. Feel the anorectal angle posteriorly. It should feel like a shelf. Ask the patient to squeeze tight and feel the difference in grip and accentuation of the angle. Poor angle or poor squeeze means damaged voluntary muscles—either directly or as a result of pudendal neuropathy: sphincter division, such as that after a third degree tear during pregnancy, may be palpable or a break in the sphincter ring. Feel for faecal masses in the rectum and also for tumours, which may interfere with the anorectal mechanism. Endoscopy may reveal proctitis, which can reduce rectal capacity.

Special tests

What may have been suspected from the history and examination can be quantified by special tests.

Manometry—This means measuring the pressure exerted on a probe in the anal canal at rest (RT) and maximal voluntary contraction (VC). RT is mainly a function of the internal sphincter. VC is wholly a function of the external sphincter and voluntary muscles. To prevent incontinence, anal pressure must always exceed intrarectal pressure.

Sensation—Patients with faecal incontinence often have an impaired ability to perceive rectal distension. This can be measured by inflating a balloon in the rectum. It may be possible to improve this ability by training.

Electromyography—Concentric needle electromyography (EMG) can be used to identify the position of the sphincter muscle in the traumatised anus, but the eye and finger are frequently as good. More sophisticated EMG techniques are at present research tools only.

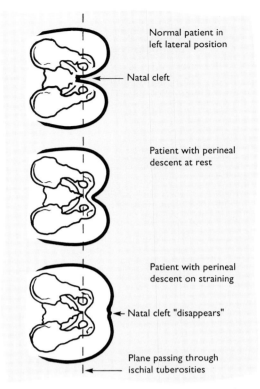

Fig 12.3 Weakness of the muscles of the pelvic floor is disclosed by a "descending perineum".

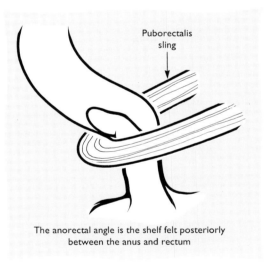

The anorectal angle is the shelf felt posteriorly between the anus and rectum

Fig 12.4 Position of anorectal angle.

Radiology—Barium enema may show a contracted rectum with a large presacral space. Defecating proctography, in which the act of defecating barium paste is observed radiologically, may provide additional information on the disorder of the defecatory mechanism such as the presence of an occult rectal prolapse. Endoanal ultrasound scanning is proving to be a simple method of demonstrating anal sphincter defects which may be amenable to surgical repair.

Treatment

Physical and social adjustments have usually been made by the time the patient presents. Indeed their unknowing friends may think them strange because they àvoid public transport and evenings out or always carry a bag or underwear and pads and keep rushing into lavatories. As in all treatment, first identify the cause. Failing that, remember that liquids are more difficult to hold than solids. Codeine phosphate or loperamide can be dramatically effective.

Rectal prolapse—In patients with rectal prolapse and faecal incontinence, rectopexy is often all that is required.

Physiotherapy—Pelvic floor exercises can be an important part of treatment provided that there is still some voluntary muscle that can be made to work. Some patients have benefited from using muscle stimulating devices for a period of some months. This works best where there is good muscle bulk, but sufficient neuropathic damage to prevent it from working naturally.

Trauma—For patients with faecal incontinence after direct obstetric or surgical trauma to the muscle, sphincter repair can be beneficial in about 85%—particularly where the surviving muscle is otherwise normal. The scar tissue is excised and an overlapping repair is made of the muscle ends to recreate a sphincter ring.

Neuropathic damage—Where faecal incontinence is the result of neuropathic damage to the pelvic floor muscles, the sphincter mechanism descends and the angle between the anal canal and rectum is lost. The operation of postanal repair seeks to recreate this angle by opposing muscle behind the rectum, thus taking it upwards and forwards. It can be successful in about half of patients.

Newer treatments are being evaluated which involve creating a new anal sphincter either from gracilis muscle in the thigh and using an implanted nerve stimulator to make it function, or using a plastic balloon device which encircles the anal canal and functions as an artificial bowel sphincter, compressing the anus.

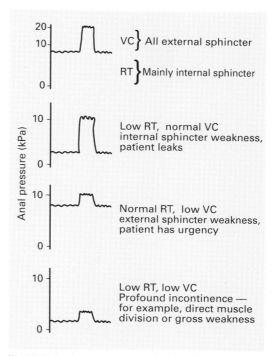

Fig 12.5 Anal manometry results showing the contributions of the internal and external sphincters to incontinence.

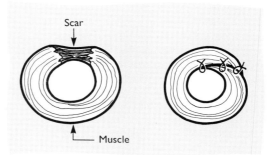

Fig 12.6 Overlapping sphincter repair gives good results in 85% of patients with traumatised sphincter.

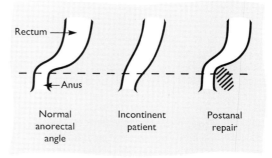

Fig 12.7 Postanal repair in patients with weakened sphincter aims to recreate the anorectal angle by reinforcing the muscle posteriorly with suture material.

13 Appendicitis

D J Jones

Appendicitis is one of the most common causes of acute abdomen in developed countries, with about one in six people undergoing appendicectomy. It is rare before the age of two years, but affects all other age groups, especially children and young adults.

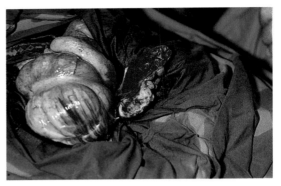
Fig 13.1 Late appendicitis.

Pathology

The clinical manifestations of acute appendicitis are the result of suppurative bacterial infection, but the aetiology is less certain. In a third of patients the appendix is obstructed by faecoliths, parasites, or lymphoid hyperplasia secondary to viral infection. The appendix is swollen, tense, congested, and lightly coated with fibrin, and the lumen is filled with purulent material. Appendicitis may resolve spontaneously, but progression to perforation and peritonitis are more likely if the appendix is not removed. The greater omentum tends to migrate to the right iliac fossa and adhere to the inflamed appendix, limiting the spread of infection and producing an inflammatory mass. Such a mass will either resolve spontaneously or progress to abscess formation with the danger of rupture into the peritoneal cavity or adjacent viscera.

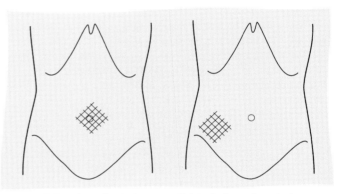
Fig 13.2 Migration of pain in appendicitis. Left: early pain is communicated through the visceral nervous system and is central in position. Right: involvement of the parietal peritoneum leads to somatic pain which is localised to the right iliac fossa.

Clinical features

About a half of patients present with a classic history of appendicitis. They develop central, constant, or colicky abdominal pain associated with anorexia, nausea, and slight vomiting. After several hours the pain migrates to the right iliac fossa. Patients appear flushed, have a tachycardia, and have a fever of up to 38·3°C, but rarely higher. They tend to lie still as movement exacerbates the pain and they have signs of localised peritonitis in the right iliac fossa. The characteristic rebound tenderness should be elicited by gentle percussion and not by the sudden release of a deeply palpating hand, which causes extreme discomfort and false positive signs. Generalised peritonitis suggests perforated appendicitis, and a tender mass

---

Conditions confused with appendicitis

Commonly
- Mesenteric adenitis
- Salpingitis
- Ectopic pregnancy
- Ruptured ovarian follicle (Mittelschmerz)
- Torsion or ruptured ovarian cyst
- Pyelonephritis and urinary tract infection
- Caecal carcinoma
- Acute cholecystitis
- Inflammatory bowel disease

Less commonly
- Perforated peptic ulcer
- Pancreatitis
- Enterocolitis
- Obstruction
- Meckel's diverticulitis
- Right lower lobe pneumonia and pleurisy
- Ureteric colic
- Shingles
- Yersinia infection
- Rectus sheath haematoma

in the right iliac fossa suggests an appendicular abscess or inflammatory mass.

Other patients do not give a classic history but experience less characteristic symptoms and signs, which vary greatly in severity. Those with an inflamed pelvic appendix may have tenderness only on rectal examination. Retrocaecal appendicitis may cause irritation and spasm of the psoas muscle, indicated by a limp and pain on hip extension. Diffuse peritonitis caused by perforation of the appendix is most common in very young and elderly patients and may not be distinguishable from other causes of generalised peritonitis.

Numerous other conditions have been mistaken for appendicitis. In children the most common difficulty is to distinguish appendicitis from mesenteric adenitis. Children with mesenteric adenitis usually have other symptoms such as sore throat and fever, which tends to be of a higher temperature than in those with acute appendicitis. Vomiting is a more prominent symptom in children, and often precedes abdominal pain and tenderness. In young women the main problem is to distinguish appendicitis from pelvic inflammatory disease, urinary tract infections, and ectopic pregnancy. A vaginal examination should be performed on reasonable suspicion of gynaecological disease; it is often difficult, however, to distinguish between tenderness resulting from salpingitis and that caused by appendicitis. In older people who develop a mass the dilemma is to distinguish appendicitis from caecal carcinoma and Crohn's disease.

Diagnosis and investigations

Appendicitis is readily diagnosed in patients presenting with classic symptoms and signs. The variable pattern of presentation in the remainder has led to inaccuracy in diagnosing acute appendicitis. Up to a third of patients undergoing surgery for suspected appendicitis have been found to have a normal appendix. The clinician's aim is to diagnose and treat appendicitis before the disease progresses to perforation and peritonitis, while at the same time avoiding unnecessary operations in those with other conditions not requiring surgery. Many investigations can be performed for patients with suspected appendicitis, but none is absolutely reliable. Efforts are now being made to diagnose appendicitis more accurately and minimise the number of unnecessary appendicectomies.

White cell count—The total white cell count is raised above 10 000/m³ in 85% of patients and three quarters have an abnormal differential white cell count, having more than 75% neutrophils. Only 4% of patients with appendicitis have both a normal white cell count and a normal neutrophil count. The white cell count, however, is raised in many other conditions, so although highly sensitive, it has poor specificity for appendicitis.

Urine analysis—This will exclude severe urinary tract infections, but an increase in the numbers of leucocytes and bacteria is often seen in acute appendicitis.

Plain abdominal radiographs—These need not be obtained in patients with suspected appendicitis. Non-specific abnormalities such as faecoliths and abnormal gas and fluid patterns may be demonstrated, but in practice these are of no help in reaching the diagnosis or deciding to operate.

Barium enema examination—This may show characteristic signs of appendicitis, including deformity, spasm, and colonic displacement. Clear filling of the appendix effectively excludes

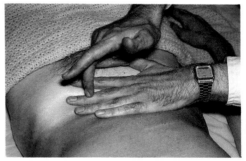

Fig 13.3 Rebound tenderness is elicited by gentle percussion and not sudden release of a deeply palpating hand.

Classic appendicitis—24 hour history

- Colicky central abdominal pain
- Anorexia
- Migration of pain to right iliac fossa
- Tachycardia
- Flushed
- Fever
- Rebound tenderness of right iliac fossa

---

appendicitis. The dose of radiation is, however, high and there is a high technical failure rate owing to inadequate imaging of the right colon.

Ultrasonography—Definite imaging of the appendix by ultrasonography is diagnostic for acute appendicitis. The sensitivity is low in those with mild appendicitis because the lumen is not sufficiently distended to obtain an image, but ultrasonography will often identify genital tract conditions in women which may be confused clinically with appendicitis.

Fine catheter aspiration—Diagnostic peritoneal aspiration using a size 14 G cannula and cytological examination may be performed to look for pus and leucocytes. It does not distinguish between appendicitis, salpingitis, and mesenteric adenitis, but if the results are negative peritoneal cytology effectively excludes all three conditions.

Laparoscopy—This is emerging as an important aid to the diagnosis of abdominal pain. It is especially valuable in young women to identify gynaecological conditions not requiring surgery. The procedure is invasive, so is indicated when surgery would otherwise be performed.

Computer aided diagnosis of abdominal pain (CADAP)—This entails obtaining the history and physical signs with reference to a structured form and the information is compared with a database to derive a probability of differential diagnoses. CADAP has improved the diagnostic accuracy for acute appendicitis and reduced the numbers of both unnecessary appendicectomies and patients with perforation in centres where it has been evaluated. Its main value is probably in directing the clinician to obtain a structured history and to elicit the relevant clinical features.

CT scanning— Recent studies show that CT scanning can be highly accurate in the diagnosis of acute appendicitis if this resource is available. The radiation dose is high and the technique should not be used routinely in young patients.

Active observation—In patients with equivocal symptoms and signs a policy of active observation and repeated examination can be pursued and appendicectomy performed if definite signs of appendicitis develop. It is extremely unlikely that patients' appendices will perforate before surgery can be performed.

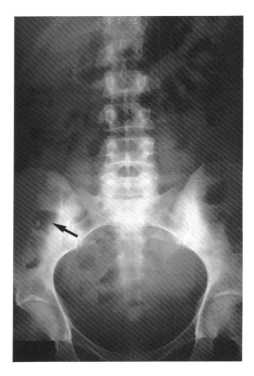

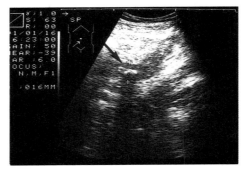

Fig 13.4 Top: plain abdominal radiograph showing a non-specific gas shadow in the right iliac fossa. Bottom: the ultrasonogram confirms a distended appendix caused by obstructing faecoliths.

Appendicectomy

Appendicectomy should be performed as soon as the patient's clinical condition permits. It is usually a relatively easy operation that is delegated to a junior surgeon; however, on occasions it may be extremely difficult. Surgery in the middle of the night is rarely indicated on clinical grounds alone.

A 5 cm transverse or oblique incision is made over the point of maximal tenderness or palpable mass in the right iliac fossa. The muscles are split lateral to the rectus abdominis. The appendicular mesentery and base of appendix are ligated and the appendix removed. Traditionally the stump is invaginated in the wall of the caecum by using a purse string suture to minimise intra-abdominal leakage and sepsis. This is probably unnecessary and is difficult if the caecum is very swollen. The peritoneal cavity is lavaged with tetracycline solution and the wound closed. Prophylactic antibiotics are given to minimise postoperative wound sepsis: a metronidazole suppository inserted preoperatively is sufficient.

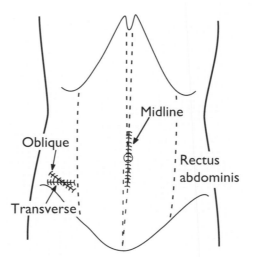

Fig 13.5 Incisions used for appendicectomy: (a) transverse at the point of maximal tenderness; (b) oblique at McBurney's point, the junction of the outer and middle thirds of a line between the anterior superior iliac spine and the umbilicus; and (c) midline when there is generalised peritonitis or doubt about the diagnosis.

The normal appendix

If the appendix proves to be normal at operation it should still be removed and the correct diagnosis sought. The right fallopian tube and ovary should be clearly visualised. The small bowel is examined for the presence of a Meckel's diverticulum; it is typically located about 0·5 m from the ileocaecal valve, but is rarely inflamed. If present, it is removed only if diseased. A number of patients prove to have terminal ileitis, which may be a manifestation of Crohn's disease. The appendix can be removed without fear of significant complications but resection of the small bowel is rarely indicated.

Incidental appendicectomy

Some surgeons remove the appendix when they perform a laparotomy for other reasons. Although this is a relatively safe procedure, complications are possible and the risk of developing appendicitis in most adults undergoing laparotomy is very small.

Appendix mass

Traditionally a policy of conservative management is adopted for patients presenting with a localised inflammatory mass. In about 80% symptoms settle, but patients require close observation in case they develop signs of spreading infection requiring surgery. Antibiotics are not given as the patient may develop an antibioma—a honeycomb of chronic abscesses. An appendix abscess can be drained percutaneously during ultrasonography. There may be a minor faecal fistula caused by the drain, but this almost invariably resolves spontaneously. Conservative management of appendicitis with antibiotics is advocated for patients in remote or inaccessible locations where surgery cannot be performed.

Patients whose condition resolves with conservative treatment should be offered an elective appendicectomy three months later to avoid further attacks. There is an emerging trend towards early appendicectomy by an experienced surgeon for patients presenting with a mass or abscess. This avoids a second hospital admission and prevents a delay in treatment for those found to have a caecal malignancy.

Laparoscopic appendicectomy

Laparoscopy already has a definite role in diagnosing lower abdominal pain, especially in young women, and removal of the appendix is an option for the experienced laparoscopic surgeon. Recovery from appendicitis may be more dependent on resolution of the disease process than on the surgical approach.

Complications

Mortality from an appendicectomy is less than 1%, but rises to 5% if the appendix is perforated, and is highest in elderly people. The principal complication is wound sepsis. This develops in about 20% of patients with perforated appendices but can be reduced to about 5% by careful surgical technique, peritoneal lavage, and antibiotic prophylaxis. If pockets of pus are not adequately drained or a haematoma develops these may develop into intra-abdominal or pelvic abscesses.

A previous appendicectomy is one of the most common causes of adhesive small bowel obstruction and one reason for minimising unnecessary appendicectomies.

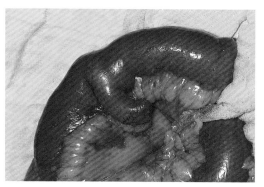
Fig 13.6 Meckel's diverticulum.

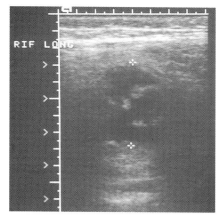
Fig 13.7 Ultrasonogram showing an appendix abscess.

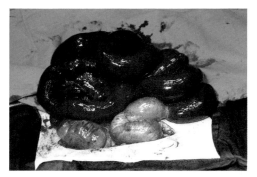
Fig 13.8 Gangrenous small bowel caused by adhesive band obstruction two years after removal of a normal appendix in a 14 year old girl.

Other related conditions

Tumours of the appendix

A carcinoid tumour is an occasional incidental finding on histological examination of the removed appendix; less commonly an adenocarcinoma is discovered. These tumours are implicated in the pathogenesis of appendicitis only on the rare occasions when they are located towards the base of the appendix and obstruct the lumen. If situated at the tip of the appendix appendicectomy will have been adequate treatment. For patients with tumours near the base of the appendix, incompletely excised tumours, or tumours greater than 2 cm in diameter, a right hemicolectomy is indicated.

Recurrent right iliac fossa pain

Recurrent right iliac fossa pain is common and often difficult to solve. In the absence of any other disease non-specific abdominal pain is diagnosed in many patients. Mild acute appendicitis can undoubtedly resolve, so recurrent attacks of appendicitis are theoretically possible and may account for the controversial diagnosis of a "grumbling appendix". In the absence of any other abnormality an appendicectomy has commonly been performed. The appendix usually appears normal both macroscopically and histologically. Although the occasional patient is relieved of pain, most continue to suffer.

> Carcinoid tumour is a rare finding on histological examination after appendicectomy. Adenocarcinoma is even less common

> Appendicectomy is rarely the answer for patients with recurrent right iliac fossa pain

14 Diverticular disease

D J Jones

Diverticula are acquired herniations of mucosa through the muscular wall of the colon. Diverticulosis indicates asymptomatic diverticular disease and diverticulitis the presence of associated inflammation.

Diverticular disease is very common in developed countries. It is associated with increasing age: it affects about a third of those over the age of 65 and half of those over 80. In 1989 in England and Wales 1480 deaths were attributed to complications of diverticular disease.

Aetiology and pathology

Diverticula are thought to arise as a pulsion phenomenon secondary to raised intraluminal pressure, which weakens the bowel wall. Constipation secondary to a low fibre diet has been implicated in this process. Muscular hypertrophy, spasm, and irregular contraction are purported to represent attempts to propel the stools in constipated patients. However, only a half of patients are constipated, so other unidentified factors must be equally important.

Diverticula are found throughout the colon but in most cases (> 90%) occur in the descending and sigmoid colon. A diverticulum consists of a pouch of mucosa covered with serosa. It herniates through the wall of the bowel at a point of natural weakness where it is penetrated by a colonic artery.

The diverticula may be large and obvious or inconspicuous, being obscured by appendices epiploicae. Viewed from within the colon they appear as slit like openings. The circular muscle coat of the bowel is thickened and the taeniae coli shortened, causing hypersegmentation of the colon.

In diverticulitis there is evidence of extramural pericolic inflammation, localised peritonitis, and, in some cases, abscess formation. Abscesses may extend to affect adjacent structures, resulting in fistulas, colovesical fistulas being the most common. Inflammation is followed by fibrosis, which occasionally causes stricturing and large bowel obstruction.

Bleeding arises when the weakened wall of a blood vessel ruptures as it passes through the wall of a diverticulum in a submucous plane. Haemorrhage may be brisk but usually stops spontaneously owing to vessel thrombosis. Traditional teaching is that diverticular disease is a common cause of lower gastrointestinal haemorrhage, but many such cases are now recognised to be caused by colonic angiodysplasia.

Diverticular disease is not a premalignant condition, but, as it is so common, it often coexists with colorectal cancers.

Clinical features

Asymptomatic diverticular disease

Many patients have incidental asymptomatic diverticular disease on endoscopy, on barium enema examination, or at operation. Probably less than a quarter of those with diverticular disease actually develop related symptoms.

Symptomatic diverticular disease

Patients with uncomplicated diverticular disease have symptoms of an irritable colon, owing to spasm and disordered

---

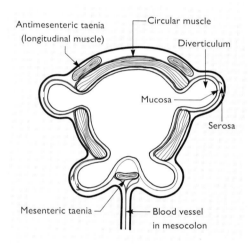

Cardinal clinical features of diverticular disease
Diverticulosis
None
Colicky pain
Altered bowel habit
Acute diverticulitis
Constant pain
Fever
Nausea and vomiting
Bleeding
Altered bowel habit
Localised or generalised tenderness

Fig 14.1 Cross section of the colon showing diverticular disease.

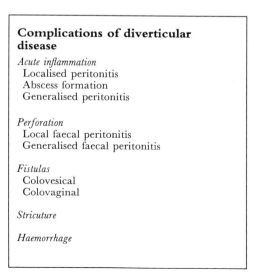

Complications of diverticular disease
Acute inflammation
Localised peritonitis
Abscess formation
Generalised peritonitis
Perforation
Local faecal peritonitis
Generalised faecal peritonitis
Fistulas
Colovesical
Colovaginal
Stricture
Haemorrhage

motility. They experience colicky pain, usually in the lower or central abdomen, associated with flatulence, distension, and altered bowel habit.

Complicated diverticular disease

Patients with acute diverticulitis experience constant pain localised to the left iliac fossa, which lasts for several days and is associated with fever and signs of local or, occasionally, diffuse peritonitis. A small proportion of patients suffer perforation and present with severe, diffuse peritonitis. Large bowel obstruction may arise secondary to a fibrous diverticular stricture or occlusion of the lumen secondary to an acute infective complication. The symptoms are rarely as severe as those of malignant large bowel obstruction.

Patients with bleeding in diverticular disease experience a sudden urge to defecate followed by the passage of a large bloody stool. This may be repeated, but bleeding usually stops spontaneously.

The most common fistula in patients with diverticular disease is between the colon and bladder. Patients with colovesical fistulas experience pneumaturia, have recurrent urinary tract infections, and pass varying amounts of faeces in the urine. Fistulas to the uterus and vagina cause a faeculant vaginal discharge.

Investigation

The mainstay of diagnosis is either a double contrast barium enema examination or colonoscopy, although both investigations may be required for full evaluation. It is often difficult to distinguish between diverticular and malignant strictures radiologically, whereas complete colonoscopy may be difficult if the colon is narrow and tortuous. Some patients have numerous large diverticular openings close together, which makes it difficult to distinguish the true lumen of the colon.

Fistulas are most easily demonstrated by barium enema examination as the site is rarely identified at colonoscopy. Limited barium studies play an important part in the investigation and diagnosis of patients with acute diverticulitis and diverticular abscess, in whom colonoscopy is associated with a significant risk of bowel perforation. Ultrasonography is useful in identifying diverticular abscesses.

Computed tomography with oral contrast is emerging as a useful method of investigating patients with suspected complicated diverticular disease. Characteristic thickening of the bowel wall may be confirmed, and the presence of associated abscess or extravasation of contrast from the colon noted.

Treatment

Diverticular disease

Dietary manipulation is the mainstay of treatment for uncomplicated diverticular disease. Patients should be advised to take a high fibre diet supplemented with a bulking agent such as bran or ispaghula to ease constipation. Pain due to muscular spasm is relieved with an antispasmodic drug such as mebeverine. The role of surgery in uncomplicated diverticular disease is small and controversial, but some patients with intractable symptoms benefit from colonic resection. Sigmoid myotomy, which involves division of the circular muscle coat of the affected colon, was once popular but carries the risk of missed perforation and has largely been abandoned.

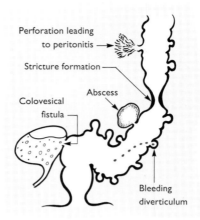

Fig 14.2 Complications of diverticular disease.

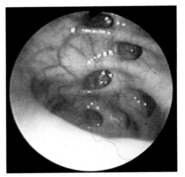

Fig 14.3 Colonoscopic view of the sigmoid colon showing diverticular openings.

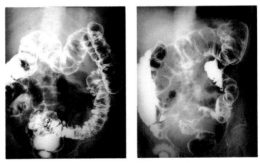

Fig 14.4 Barium enema radiographs showing uncomplicated diverticular disease (left) and a diverticular stricture (right). This is difficult to distinguish from cancer; colonoscopy is essential.

Treatment of diverticular disease

Uncomplicated	—High fibre diet —Bulk laxative —Antispasmodics	*Perforation*	—Laparotomy —Peritoneal lavage —Antibiotics —Possible resection —Possible delayed anastomosis
Severe uncomplicated	—Colectomy	*Fistula*	—Elective resection —Primary anastomosis
Diverticulitis	—Intravenous fluids —Broad spectrum antibiotics	*Haemorrhage*	—Resuscitation —Colectomy (if life threatening)
Abscess	—Percutaneous drainage	*Obstruction*	—Resection with delayed or primary anastomosis depending on circumstances

Acute diverticulits

The mainstay of treatment for acute diverticulitis is rest, analgesia, broad spectrum antibiotics, and either oral or intravenous fluids depending on the patient's general condition. Most patients settle on this treatment and surgery is not necessary. After recovery from an acute attack of diverticulitis, patients are treated as for uncomplicated diverticular disease. If a patient is subjected to laparotomy and discovered to have acute diverticulitis antibiotics should be administered, the peritoneal cavity lavaged with tetracycline solution, and the abdomen closed. Colonic resection or the creation of a transverse loop colostomy are not necessary for localised diverticulitis. A minority of patients with acute diverticulitis do not respond to conservative treatment and develop diffuse peritonitis or local abscesses requiring surgical intervention.

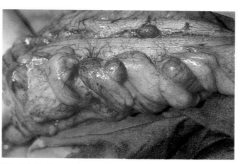

Fig 14.5 Operative photograph of diverticular disease in the sigmoid colon.

Diverticular abscess

Most diverticular abscesses are now confirmed by ultrasonography or computed tomography and can be drained percutaneously. Abscesses can also be drained at open operation, but care is essential to avoid contamination of the peritoneal cavity with pus and faeces. A defunctioning colostomy is not necessary. Many patients will develop a faecal fistula via the drain site, but the discharge is usually slight and most close spontaneously in the absence of distal obstruction.

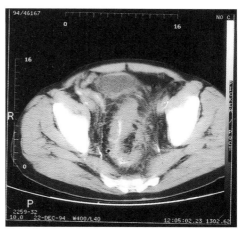

Fig 14.6 Contrast CT scan showing inflammatory phlegmon in severe acute diverticulitis.

Generalised peritonitis

A laparotomy is performed for generalised peritonitis, pus and faeces removed, and the peritoneal cavity thoroughly lavaged with tetracycline solution. Further progression of sepsis is prevented by resection of the diseased segment of colon.

A transverse loop colostomy without resection was once popular, but this does not effectively defunction the diseased segment, because faeces tend to spill over into the distal colon, preventing resolution of the sepsis. Resection removes the diseased bowel and provides an opportunity for histological confirmation of the diagnosis as confident distinction between diverticular disease and malignancy is often difficult at operation.

Primary anastomosis in the unprepared colon, which may be loaded with faeces, in the presence of sepsis carries a risk of anastomotic leakage and breakdown. The preferred operation is to resect the diseased bowel, exteriorising the proximal colon as an end colostomy, and either closing over the distal large bowel with sutures (Hartmann's procedure) or exteriorising it as a non-functioning mucus fistula. Continuity of the large bowel is restored at a later date when the patient has fully recovered. Resection of complicated diverticular disease and reversal of a Hartmann's procedure are often technically demanding and should be performed by an experienced surgeon.

Diverticular fistulas

Traditionally, diverticular fistulas were defunctioned by a proximal transverse loop colostomy, allowing resolution of inflammation at the site of the fistula, hence facilitating subsequent staged resection and closure. With adequate bowel preparation and prophylactic antibiotics, it is often possible to perform a single operation with resection of the diseased colon and repair of the fistula.

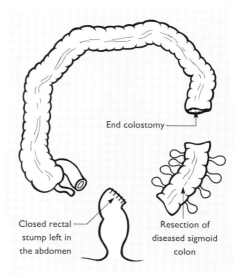

End colostomy

Closed rectal stump left in the abdomen

Resection of diseased sigmoid colon

Fig 14.7 Hartmann's procedure.

Diverticular haemorrhage

Most patients with bleeding in association with diverticular disease settle on conservative management, but resection is occasionally necessary for life threatening haemorrhage. Radionuclide imaging and arteriography may help in localising the source of haemorrhage and identifying bleeding caused by angiodysplasias. If the site of bleeding is identified a segmental resection is performed. If the site can not be determined preoperatively or during surgery subtotal colectomy and ileorectal anastomosis may be necessary.

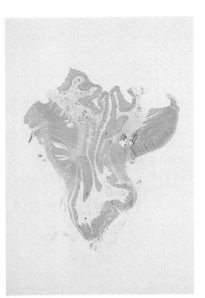

Fig 14.9 Histological slide of a diverticulum showing herniation of mucosa through the muscular layer of the wall of the colon.

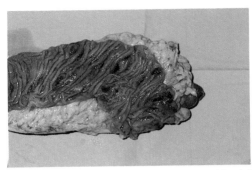

Fig 14.8 Pathological photograph showing blood filled diverticular pits in a colon removed because of major lower gastrointestinal haemorrhage thought to be the result of diverticular disease.

15 Inflammatory bowel disease

N A Scott, D G Thompson

Non-specific inflammatory bowel disease includes Crohn's disease, ulcerative colitis, and indeterminate colitis. Each condition is defined by its distribution, clinical behaviour, and/or histological characteristics (Table 15.1). Medical and surgical management of inflammatory bowel disease is directed at symptoms only because there continues to be a lack of understanding as to the underlying cause(s) of these diseases.

Ulcerative colitis

Aetiology and incidence

New cases of ulcerative colitis are seen at a rate of 10–15 new cases per 100 000 of the population each year. Overall the prevalence of this condition is about 60 cases per 100 000 of the population. A positive family history might be expected in about 10% of patients with ulcerative colitis. Changes in faecal flora, a history of non-smoking, milk allergy, and an autoimmune response have all been considered as important in the aetiology of ulcerative colitis. The primary pathological process remains, however, unknown.

Clinical features

The clinical severity of ulcerative colitis is extremely variable. For most patients, passage of frequent stools that are blood stained and with mucus is the most common initial presentation. In addition some patients complain of mild lower abdominal pain and tenesmus, but have little in the way of systemic upset or weight loss. Abdominal examination is usually unremarkable but rectal examination reveals blood and, on unprepared rigid sigmoidoscopy, there is evidence of proctitis. Biopsy of the rectal mucosa is performed to confirm the diagnosis histologically.

A minority of patients with ulcerative colitis present either initially or subsequently with a severe attack of colitis. Such a patient has unremitting bloody diarrhoea (10–24 times a day), colicky lower abdominal pain, and weight loss. On examination the patient looks pale and ill, and has tachycardia, pyrexia, and a tender lower abdomen.

Imaging in chronic ulcerative colitis

Colonoscopy is the definitive technique for imaging the colon in chronic ulcerative colitis. The elective outpatient is prepared in the usual way and a full examination to the caecum is performed. In many patients the macroscopic distribution of the colitis is confined to the rectum and part of the sigmoid colon in continuity. Systematic biopsies throughout the colon enable diagnosis, definition of distribution, and identification of dysplasia. A barium enema is used less frequently in the imaging of ulcerative colitis but it can be used for identifying the characteristic distribution of ulcerative colitis.

Management

The management of all patients with inflammatory bowel disease is the management of symptoms. This requires an integrated medical and surgical approach that delivers the appropriate therapy consistent with symptom relief.

Table 15.1. Characteristics of ulcerative colitis, Crohn's disease, and indeterminate colitis

Characteristic	Ulcerative colitis	Crohn's disease	Indeterminate colitis
Distribution	Colon	All gastrointestinal tract	Colon
Gut involved	Mucosa only	All layers	Mucosa to muscularis
Histology	Crypt abscess	Non-caseating granuloma	
	Goblet cell mucin depletion	Fissuring ulcer	

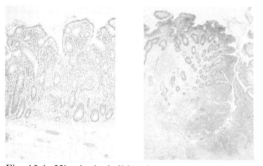

Fig. 15.1. Histological slides showing ulcerative colitis (left) confined to the mucosa and small bowel in Crohn's disease (right) with transmural inflammation fissuring ulcer.

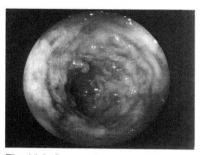

Fig. 15.2. Severe ulcerative colitis viewed through a colonoscope.

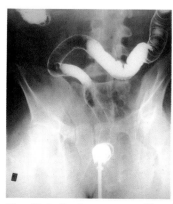

Fig. 15.3. Barium enema film showing a hosepipe colon in chronic ulcerative colitis.

Medical management — Management of the stable patient consists of drug therapy (proctitis: steroid or mesalazine enemas; colitis: oral prednisolone, mesalazine) at a minimum dose that is compatible with good health and the fewest side effects. Such a patient may be maintained for months or years on minimal medication, with occasional periods of high dose steroid therapy for exacerbations of colitic symptoms. Colonoscopic surveillance, once every three years, for evidence of mucosal dysplasia is usually started 10 years after the diagnosis. A long history of colitis and a pancolitic distribution of disease are both associated with the potential for malignant change in the colonic mucosa. Mucosal biopsies that show high grade dysplasia or carcinoma in situ indicate the need for surgical removal of the colon to prevent the development of invasive colon cancer.

Toxic 'disintegrative' colitis — A few patients with ulcerative colitis present with or develop an acute exacerbation of their colitic symptoms that fails to respond quickly to oral high dose steroids taken as an outpatient. Such patients require treatment in hospital as inpatients. An initial assessment is made of abdominal tenderness, stool frequency, temperature, and pulse rate. Investigations include full blood count, erythrocyte sedimentation rate (ESR), serum albumin, acute phase proteins (C reactive protein [CRP] and orosomucoids), and plain abdominal radiology. Intravenous fluids and hydrocortisone 100 mg three times daily, with bed rest, forms the mainstay of medical therapy for an acute exacerbation of colitis.

Combined medical and surgical management from admission is critical for such patients, because failure to respond quickly to medical measures is an indication for abdominal colectomy. In the patient who does not respond to medical therapy, the colon is in the process of disintegration. This means that it is a catastrophic error to delay surgery until there is evidence of toxic dilatation. Once it is clear that medical therapy has not arrested the exacerbation within 72 hours of admission, then it is the role of both the surgeon and the physician to persuade the patient of the need for colectomy. In the acutely ill patient the surgical procedure comprises abdominal colectomy, end ileostomy, and preservation of the rectum with a mucus fistula.

Subsequent removal of the rectum will be necessary in most patients for surgical cure of ulcerative colitis. With male patients it is important to discuss the small but definite risk of impotence that can result from proctectomy. Dissection techniques that stay close to the rectal wall minimise the chances of pelvic autonomic nerve injury.

Restorative surgery: the pouch — The elimination of ulcerative colitis, and any associated risk of cancer, can be achieved by the removal of all colonic mucosa. Thus, the operation of panproctocolectomy was, for many years, the "gold standard" procedure for curing ulcerative colitis — the principal disadvantage being a permanent end ileostomy. By contrast, the ileal pouch (J, W or S pouch), or the construction of a new reservoir or neorectum to replace the removed diseased rectum offers the chance of surgical cure for ulcerative colitis and indeterminate colitis, without the need for a permanent ileostomy. The ileoanal pouch is now the reconstructive operation of choice in patients with ulcerative colitis and indeterminate colitis, but it is contraindicated in Crohn's disease (see below).

A most important aspect of restorative pouch surgery is repeated detailed discussions with the patient about what the pouch procedure does and does not offer. The surgeon and the specialised colorectal nurse must explain that the ileal pouch

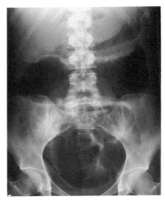

Fig. 15.4. Abdominal radiograph showing toxic dilation in disintegrative colitis.

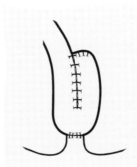

Fig. 15.5. Duplicated ileoanal pouch (J pouch). The reservoir is constructed by joining together two adjacent lengths of ileum. It is then anastomosed to the anal canal.

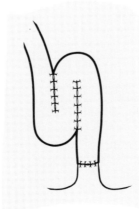

Fig. 15.6. Triplicated ileoanal pouch (Park's pouch). A larger reservoir is produced by joining together three adjacent lengths of ileum.

does not offer the patient the "normal" bowel function that they enjoyed before the onset of colitis. It is important that the surgeon's own *local* results of pouch surgery, stool frequency, incidence of incontinence, and rate of pouch failure and excision are included in the discussion with the prospective pouch patient.

The ileal reservoir most commonly employed is the J pouch, which is constructed from about 40 cm of distal ileum and stapled or sutured onto the anal canal, so that pouch continence is maintained by the anal sphincter. The newly constructed pouch is usually defunctioned by a loop ileostomy for three months. In very favourable circumstances, the loop ileostomy may be dispensed with; however, its omission places the patient at risk from severe pelvic sepsis and even death if there is a pouch leak. Three months after pouch construction, a contrast study of the pouch is performed to confirm that the suture line of the pouch is intact, in which case the loop ileostomy is closed. Frequency of pouch evacuation usually settles at 4–5 times/day with good continence, assisted by the constipating agents loperamide and codeine phosphate which slow intestinal transit.

Crohn's disease

Aetiology and incidence

Crohn's disease is a transmural inflammatory bowel disease which can affect any part of the gastrointestinal tract, from the mouth to the anus. The incidence of Crohn's disease is about three new cases per 100 000 with a prevalence of about 30 cases per 100 000 of the population. Environmental and genetic factors are both implicated in the causation of Crohn's disease. About 10% of patients with Crohn's disease give a positive family history of inflammatory bowel disease. Infective agents, about which there is speculation about their role as aetiological agents, include the measles virus and *Mycobacterium paratuberculosis*. There have been consistent reports of increased sugar consumption in populations of patients with Crohn's disease when compared with controls. The aetiological factor that could provide a preventative or curative strategy remains elusive, however.

Clinical features

Patients with Crohn's disease are usually young (peak 15–35 years) and female, and present with abdominal pain, weight loss, and diarrhoea. For many patients the cause of these symptoms may not be established for some time after their onset. Symptoms can progress to subacute small bowel obstruction as a result of a Crohn's stricture of the terminal ileum. The abdominal pain is colicky, associated with loud borborygmi and distension, often precipitated by a meal eaten 30 minutes before. Such patients learn to avoid solid indigestible food and may initiate their own low residue diet to avoid attacks of pain. The presence of an abdominal mass, usually in the right iliac fossa, suggests the possibility of fistulating Crohn's disease with formation of an inflammatory mass and/or abscess. If the abscess discharges onto the skin, an enterocutaneous fistula is produced. Discharge of the abscess into an adjacent viscus produces internal fistulation — enteroenteric, enterovesical, and enterocolonic. Extraintestinal manifestations of Crohn's disease include erythema nodosum, pyoderma gangrenosum, uveitis and sacroileitis, large joint involvement, and clubbing.

A minority of patients with Crohn's disease present with the symptoms of colitis: frequent bloody stools with mucus. These patients are indistinguishable from those with ulcerative colitis, including the occasional development of toxic colitis. Perianal Crohn's disease (PCD) is a feature of about 7% of patients with

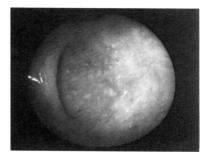
Fig. 15.7. Mild ulcerative colitis viewed through a colonoscope

Incidence of Crohn's disease from surveys		
Country	Incidence (cases/ 100 000 population)	Years studied
North east Scotland	4·6	1962-8
Malmö, Sweden	6·0	1966-8
United States	4·5	1973
Cardiff, Wales	4·9	1976-80
Copenhagen, Denmark	2·7	1970-8

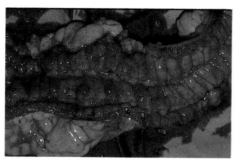
Fig. 15.8. Pathological specimen of opened colon showing Crohn's colitis with deep fissuring, giving a cobblestoned appearance.

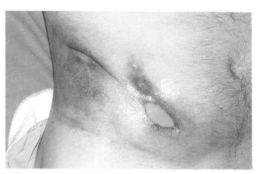
Fig. 15.9. Severe manifestations of Crohn's disease with multiple enterocutaneous fistulas.

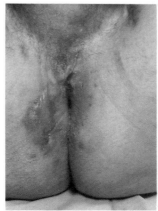
Fig. 15.10. Watering can perineum with multiple perianal fistulas.

Crohn's disease. It is often associated with colonic disease, but can also be seen with small bowel disease or even in isolation. Perianal pain and suppuration are the main symptoms in the patient with PCD. Rectal examination reveals evidence of ulceration, oedematous skin tags, perianal abscess/fistulation, and stricture.

Imaging

Crohn's disease can be detected by demonstration of bowel wall thickening in the right iliac fossa on ultrasonography. For diagnostic purposes a small bowel enema is, however, preferable and probably superior to a barium meal and follow through. Characteristic findings include aphthous ulcers, long strictures (string sign of Kantor), fissuring ulceration, fistulation, and skip lesions. Intra-abdominal abscess formation can be detected by ultrasonography but computed tomography is often more accurate.

Colonic disease is best diagnosed by colonoscopy. The distribution of colitis is discontinuous with rectal sparing. Often the terminal ileum can be visualised and biopsied to confirm small bowel disease. Barium enema examination will also demonstrate Crohn's colitis and reflux of barium into the terminal ileum can be used to diagnose disease at this site. White cell scans, using technetium labelled white cells, can also be useful in delineating the distribution of inflammatory bowel disease.

Definitive imaging of perianal disease may require examination under anaesthetic with endoscopy of the rectum. Other techniques that might help in defining perianal lesions include transrectal ultrasonography and magnetic resonance imaging of the anal canal.

Management

Medical management — The aim of management is symptom relief and maintenance of wellbeing, with the minimum of side effects associated with the treatment and dose. It is also important for the patient to have a balanced diet and to maintain weight. An acute flareup of obstructive symptoms can be managed by a short high dose regimen of oral prednisolone 30–40 mg/day for two weeks, rapidly reducing the dose to a smaller maintenance dose of 5–10 mg/day over six weeks. In the patient with Crohn's disease in whom oral steroids cannot be reduced below an acceptable level without symptom reactivation, azathioprine may allow maintenance at a lower steroid dosage. Budesonide is a newer preparation of enteric coated steroid which is released into the terminal ileum. It offers a means of treating small bowel Crohn's disease without the systemic side effects of conventional oral steroids, because the drug is largely removed on its passage through the liver.

Crohn's disease activity can be monitored through measurement of the haemoglobin, the platelet count, ESR, CRP, and orosomucoids. In the patient with quiescent colonic disease suphasalazine derivatives may also be used (for example, mesalazine or pentasa).

Surgical management — Experience suggests that the understandable fear of surgery delays the first surgical removal of symptomatic Crohn's disease. Integrated medical and surgical management is required in practice to achieve the correct use of surgical resection as treatment. Surgery is used in Crohn's disease when drug therapy cannot achieve optimal relief of symptoms with an acceptable level of side effects (for example, in steroids, these are osteoporosis, acne, hypertension and cushingoid facies). The presence of a mass in association with Crohn's disease is an absolute indication for operation.

Preoperative counselling should address the principal fears of the patient with Crohn's disease. These include the risk of a

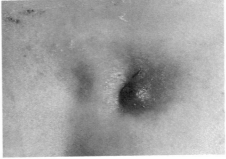

Fig. 15.11. Crohn's enterocutaneous fistulas emerging in lumbrosacral arc.

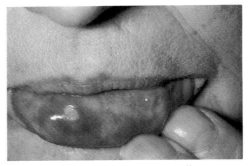

Fig. 15.12. Mouth ulcers in Crohn's disease.

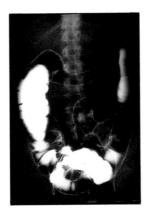

Fig. 15.13.

stoma and the need for repeated surgery. Most resections for obstructing terminal ileal disease will be followed by reanastomosis and do not require an ileostomy. By contrast, patients who are malnourished with sepsis from an abscess or fistula may require exteriorisation of the intestine. In most such patients, however, reanastomosis of exteriorised bowel would be undertaken 3–6 months later. Future surgery for recrudescence of Crohn's disease might be necessary for about 50% of patients over the course of a 10 year follow up period.

The guiding principle in surgical resection of Crohn's disease is to inspect the entire small bowel and remove only the disease that is the cause of the patient's symptoms. In the large majority, this means resection of a length (perhaps 30 cm) of terminal ileum, and the caecum or the ileocolonic anastomosis. By contrast, the neglect of a Crohn's mass leads to fistulation into adjacent normal loops of bowel, which in turn can result in a much more extensive small bowel resection. Involvement of the sigmoid colon by fistulating terminal ileal disease, or of the duodenum by fistulation from an ileocolonic anastomosis, can further increase the complexity of the surgical procedure.

Diffuse stricturing Crohn's disease of the small bowel is less commonly encountered. Surgical exploration of the gut through an enterotomy with a Foley catheter balloon distended to 2·5 cm diameter will identify the strictures responsible for mechanical obstruction. If the strictures are closely grouped over a limited length of small bowel, resection of that length and anastomosis are quite acceptable. Strictureplasty, longitudinal division of the Crohn's stricture with transverse resuture, is reserved for the small minority of patients who have had either extensive small bowel resection or multiple widely separated Crohn's strictures — resection of which would risk the short bowel syndrome.

Patients with Crohn's colitis come to surgery because of chronic ill health, but they can also present acutely with a disintegrative colitis requiring urgent colectomy. The tendency of Crohn's colitis to spare the rectum means that ileorectal anastomosis is the preferred option for subsequent reconstruction. Segmental Crohn's colitis also lends itself to segmental resection and reanastomosis. Many patients with Crohn's colitis will require panproctocolectomy to eliminate their colonic symptoms. The ileal pouch is *not* a generally accepted option after colectomy for Crohn's colitis, because of the propensity of Crohn's disease to affect the pouch, leading to its failure and subsequent removal. Patients need to be informed of the small risk of autonomic nerve damage and non-healing perineal sinus that can follow proctectomy.

Perianal Crohn's disease

Perianal pain and suppuration in Crohn's disease herald the development of perianal Crohn's lesions. Typically, a fissuring ulcer in the anal canal leads to abscess formation and then fistulation to the perianal skin or the vagina. Aggressive surgical drainage of sepsis has to be tempered by the need to preserve sphincter function if a permanent stoma is to be avoided. Long term oral metronidazole (accompanied by warnings of peripheral neuropathy) can reduce the severity and the frequency of perianal sepsis in some patients.

Anal pain without suppuration caused by a fissuring ulcer in the anal canal can be helped by an injection of methylprednisolone (Depo-Medrone) into the ulcer. Drainage of perianal abscesses is necessary when they occur. Low superficial fistulas can be layed open, but healing can be unpredictable. Drainage of trans-sphincteric and higher fistulas is best achieved by a seton — usually a polypropylene (Prolene) suture inserted through the length of the fistula and tied loosely. Such measures can alleviate perianal symptoms and allow an acceptable quality of life without a stoma. Failure of these measures leads initially to a defunctioning stoma; this

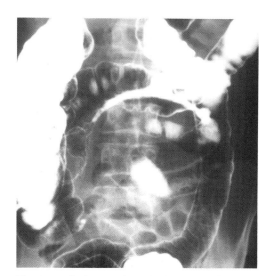

Fig. 15.14. Stricture of terminal ileum in Crohn's disease.

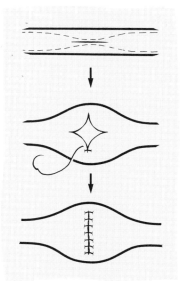

Fig. 15.15. Small bowel with multiple strictures.

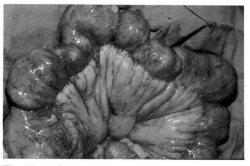

Fig. 15.16. Strictureplasty. The narrow segment of bowel affected in Crohn's disease is opened longitudinally. The opening is then closed transversely to increase the size of the lumen.

reduces perianal symptoms but rarely results in complete resolution of the perianal Crohn's lesions.

Subsequent closure of the loop stoma is often followed by reactivation of the perianal symptoms and may pave the way to consideration of proctectomy. Stricture of the anal canal can be the principal cause of a patient's symptoms, but is usually seen in association with ulcer and fistula. Dilation under an anaesthetic, coupled with regular self dilatation thereafter, can result in reasonable symptom relief.

Perianal Crohn's disease in women can progress to involve the vagina by fistulation. In most patients, a low fistula communicates from the anal sphincter into the lower vagina. Symptoms consist of a minimal purulent discharge which often does not require any specific therapy other than reassurance. More persistent symptoms from an anovaginal connection, which fail to settle on metronidazole treatment or insertion of a seton, may warrant repair with flap advancement. By contrast, a Crohn's rectovaginal fistula involves a much larger communication between the vagina and the rectum, resulting in frank faecal incontinence through the vagina. The rectovaginal fistula has a much poorer prognosis; a defunctioning stoma and/or an advancement flap may be attempted but proctectomy is a strong possibility in affected women.

Inflammatory bowel disease: the team

The characteristic feature of a diagnosis of inflammatory bowel disease, for a patient, is *uncertainty*: uncertainty about cause, prognosis, treatment, continence, personal relationships, fertility, education, employment, surgery, stoma, and cancer. Living with an uncertainty of this magnitude causes considerable distress and fear for many patients with inflammatory bowel disease. Good relevant patient information, both locally based and via national organisations, is critical in informing the individual patient about future possibilities and giving crucial quantification of the likelihood of these outcomes. A major priority of the medical and nursing staff should be to give the patient control over his or her symptoms, treatment, and future. This aim requires both time and commitment from the clinician, in order to explain the implications of the disease and medical and surgical therapy; this is probably best delivered in a specialist clinic supported by nurses experienced in the management of inflammatory bowel disease.

Teamwork is the expression used to encourage close integration of medical and surgical gastroenterology, to optimise therapeutic options available to the patient with inflammatory bowel disease. In reality, the medical professionals are merely the managers and coaches on the sideline — the only "team" on the pitch is the patient.

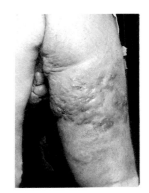

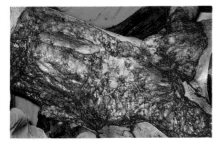

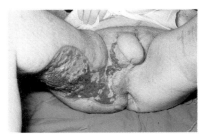

Fig. 15.17. (Top) Extensive perianal Crohn's disease extending into the thigh. (Middle) The diseased skin has been excised down to the deep fascia. (Bottom) Healing perineum and thigh after skin mesh grafting.

Useful support groups

National Association for Colitis and Crohn's disease (NACC)
PO Box 205
St Albans
Herts AL1 1AB

Ileostemy and Internal Pouch Support Group
PO Box 23
Mansfield
Notts NG18 4TT

British Digestive Foundation
3 St Andrew's Place
London NW1 4LB

16 Colorectal Neoplasia—I: Benign colonic tumours

D J Jones

The term "polyp" is often wrongly used synonymously with "benign colonic tumour". A polyp is a descriptive term for a pedunculated lesion. Not all polyps are tumours; not all polypoid tumours are benign and not all benign tumours are polypoid.

Benign tumours can be classified into those of epithelial origin, those of mesodermal origin, and hamartomas.

Mesodermal tumours

Mesodermal tumours are usually sessile but may be polypoid. Lipoma and leiomyoma are not uncommon in postmortem material but are rarely symptomatic. If symptoms occur it is usually because of ulceration in the overlying mucosa with bleeding. Rarely they may cause intussusception.

Haemangioma

True haemangiomas are very rare but may cause life threatening bleeding. They should be distinguished from angiodysplasia—small telangiectatic lesions that occur in elderly people. These are too small to be diagnosed by any means other than colonoscopy or angiography; they are one of the causes of massive colonic bleeding.

Hamartoma

Juvenile polyp

Juvenile polyps are the most common polyps in children. They are histologically distinct from other polyps and can occur anywhere in the large bowel but are most common in the rectum. They occur in girls and boys usually below the age of 10 years and may be familial.

They present with either prolapse through the anus or bleeding as a result of ulceration or autoamputation. They are not premalignant and may be treated by local endoscopic resection.

Peutz–Jeghers syndrome

Peutz-Jeghers syndrome is a rare disease which is usually familial. It causes pigmentation around the lips associated with characteristic intestinal polyps. The polyps are most common in the small intestine, though they can occur in the stomach or colon.

The microscopic appearance of the polyps is of a coralline arrangement of muscularis mucosa covered with epithelium. They often first present in childhood with intussusception or bleeding. The polyps have a low grade malignant potential. Treatment is difficult because of the widespread nature of the polyps and is confined to surgery to deal with the serious complications.

Epithelial tumours

Metaplastic (hyperplastic) polyps and adenomas

It is important to distinguish metaplastic polyps from true adenomas. Metaplastic polyps are tiny plaques of hyperplastic epithelium 1–2 mm in size. They are not premalignant and can be safely left alone.

Adenomas are premalignant lesions, although the risk of

Classification of large bowel polyps
Epithelial
Adenoma: tubular; tubulovillous; villous
Metaplastic polyp
Mesodermal
Lipoma
Leiomyoma
Haemangioma
Other rare tumours
Hamartoma
Juvenile polyps
Peutz–Jeghers polyp

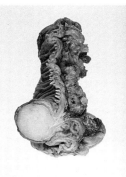

Fig 16.1 Large lipoma arising at the ileocaecal valve.

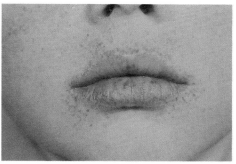

Fig 16.2 Facial features of Peutz–Jeghers syndrome.

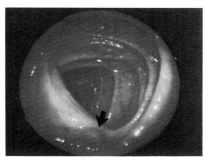

Fig 16.3 Metaplastic polyp viewed through a colonoscope.

malignant transformation for an individual adenoma is low. The risk of malignancy inceases with the size of the adenoma, and villous adenomas are more prone to malignant transformation than tubular adenomas.

Tubular adenomas are commonly multiple and may coexist with a carcinoma. The possibility of coincident carcinoma is greater when the polyps are multiple. They may be asymptomatic or cause bleeding, prolapse, or intussusception.

Familial adenomatous polyposis

Familial adenomatous polyposis is an autosomal dominant condition caused by a germ line mutation of the adenomatous polyposis (APC) gene located on the long arm of chromosome 5 in band q 21. About 25% of cases are caused by new mutations and such patients do not give a family history. The affected colon is carpeted with hundreds of polyps. The disease develops in early adult life and inevitably undergoes malignant transformation about 10 years after onset. Patients often have other abnormalities, including multiple osteomas, epidermoid cysts, fibrous tumours, and periampullary tumours in the duodenum. These extracolonic manifestations are most prominent in Gardner's syndrome, which is now considered to be part of the spectrum of familial adenomatous polyposis.

Diagnosis of adenomas

Most adenomas are asymptomatic. An adenoma may be discovered incidentally when the colon is being investigated for a symptomatic lesion or as a result of a health screening programme. More than 10% of the population aged over 45 years might have asymptomatic adenomas.

Symptoms may be bleeding or prolapse of the polyp through the anus, or, rarely, intussusception. Diarrhoea or discharge of mucus occurs in patients with multiple polyps or, typically, in those with villous adenoma. Extreme potassium loss from a villous adenoma may result in hypokalaemia, but this is rare.

Many adenomas are either palpable by rectal examination or easily seen on sigmoidoscopy. Total colonoscopy is the best investigation for detecting adenomas, but high quality double contrast barium enema examination is almost as good.

When an adenoma is discovered it is important to ask, "Has it undergone malignant transformation?" If the tumour is palpable, hard areas suggest malignancy, as does ulceration of the polyps seen on endoscopy. Large tumours are more likely to be malignant. Finally, tumours shown to be villous on histological examination are more commonly associated with malignancy.

The second question must be, "Is the adenoma solitary?" It is well known that adenomas may be multiple and associated with large bowel cancer at another site. A full investigation of the whole colon is essential.

Treatment of adenomas

Solitary adenomas

Many adenomas are pedunculated and can be removed after ligation of the pedicle, either directly after prolapsing the tumour through the anus or by snare diathermy through a sigmoidoscope or colonoscope.

A small sessile lesion can be snared or excised in the submucosal plane or destroyed by hot diathermy forceps through the colonoscope. A large sessile lesion in the rectum can be destroyed by diathermy or submucous dissection, but dealing with large sessile polyps colonoscopically may be hazardous.

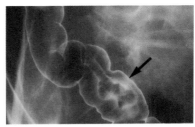
Fig 16.4 Barium enema radiograph showing a colonic adenoma.

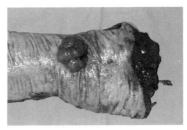
Fig 16.5 Colonic adenoma.

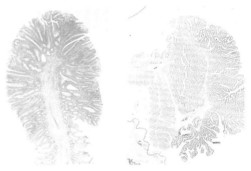
Fig 16.6 Histological slides showing tubular adenoma (left) and villous adenoma (right).

Symptoms of tubular adenoma

- None
- Bleeding
- Prolapse
- Intrussusception

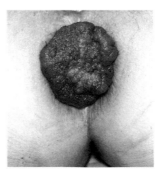
Fig 16.7 Villous adenoma prolapsing through the anus.

Complete excision biopsy is desirable for good pathological assessment, and for this reason diathermy destruction is less satisfactory. If the pathologist discovers carcinoma in the polyp but without invasion up to the line of resection, then no further action is required. If the line of section is involved, surgery, as for carcinoma, is indicated.

In moderately sized sessile or large tumours (> 5 cm), surgical excision is probably the safest option. At operation a colotomy and local excision or a small segmental resection can be used. Polyps in the rectum can be removed through the anus or by the trans-sacral approach.

Once a patient has been rendered free of polyps, he or she should be offered repeat colonoscopy every five years because of the risk of developing further adenomas.

Familial adenomatous polyposis

Surgery is indicated in patients with familial adenomatous polyposis before malignant transformation occurs. Many patients can be identified by careful screening of families of known patients. Congenital hypertrophy of the retinal pigmented epithelium is highly specific for familial adenomatous polyposis and is easily detected on ophthalmological examination. It can be discovered before polyps develop. Affected people can also be identified with 95% confidence by DNA screening.

Total colectomy with ileorectal anastomosis, followed by regular outpatient surveillance of the residual rectum and treatment of polyps endoscopically as necessary, has commonly been used but has the disadvantage that all series contain patients in whom rectal cancer has developed. The traditional alternative is to offer panproctocolectomy which leaves the patient with a permanent ileostomy. A more recent development is to perform a restorative proctocolectomy, by constructing an ileal pouch which is anastomosed to the preserved anal canal. For patients with slight rectal involvement, it is feasible to perform an ileorectal anastomosis with a view to a completion proctectomy and permanent ileostomy or pouch once the patient has a stable working and family lifestyle.

Few patients with familial adenomatous polyposis develop cancers after they have undergone prophylactic colectomy. They require long term follow up however, because of the extracolonic manifestations, especially ampullary tumours in the duodenum and desmoid tumours, which have become the most common cause of death.

Villous tumours

Careful assessment is necessary to exclude second tumours and malignant transformation in patients with villous tumours. In the lower or mid rectum full assessment is possible and for a benign lesion local excision is appropriate. For an extensive lesion in the upper rectum or colon an appropriate colonic or rectal excision with anastomosis is indicated.

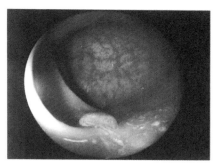

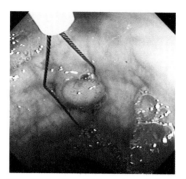

Fig. 16.8. Top: Polyp viewed through a colonoscope. Bottom: snared polyp.

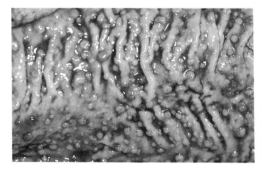

Fig. 16.9. Colon with familial adenomatous polyposis.

17 Colorectal neoplasia—II: Large bowel cancer

D Jones

Carcinoma of the large bowel is a common malignancy. It is predominantly a disease of older people, though it may occur at any age. Less than 5% of patients are under the age of 40 and more than half are over 60, with the peak incidence in people aged 70–80.

There are about 28 000 new cases each year in the United Kingdom, and it is second only to cancer of the bronchus as a cause of death from cancer, with an annual mortality of about 19 000. The overall survival rate for colorectal cancer in the United Kingdom is about 38% after five years. There is no noticeable sex difference; in women it is less common than carcinoma of the breast. There has been no significant change in mortality from large bowel cancer over the past 40 years and half the cases present beyond surgical cure.

Aetiology

Most, if not all, colorectal cancers arise from an adenoma. The risk of malignant transformation in any individual polyp is low. It increases with increasing size of the adenoma, and villous adenomas are much more prone to malignant transformation than tubular adenomas.

Colorectal tumorigenesis is considered to be a multistep process, including hyperproliferative mucosa, adenomas, and carcinomas. A combination of both environmental and genetic factors play an important part in pathogenesis.

Environmental factors

There is considerable variation world wide in the incidence of colorectal cancer. It seems to be particularly prevalent in highly developed countries, so that there is a high rate in the United Kingdom, the United States of America, Australasia, and western Europe, but a low incidence in central Africa and Asia. This geographical variation has been ascribed by many to different diets. Initially a low fibre diet was suggested as the causative factor, and subsequently an excess of animal fat or protein. Epidemiological evidence is contradictory. Part of the problem is that there are usually multiple differences in diet between different ethnic groups and it becomes difficult to know which component or components can be considered responsible. The paradox is illustrated by the Eskimos, who have a low fibre, high fat diet and a very low incidence of large bowel cancer. Dietary factors do, however, seem to play some part because when black Africans adopt a Western diet their indicence of colorectal tumours progressively increases.

It is thought that diet produces its effect through generating intraluminal carcinogens. Fibre has been propounded as a protective agent because it decreases bowel transit time, increases stool bulk, and binds intraluminal carcinogens, which reduces the contact time of any potential carcinogen with the mucosa.

A second hypothesis is that dietary alterations may alter the bacterial flora in the gut. Certain bacteria are known to degrade bile salts to form carcinogens. In epidemiological studies such bacteria and higher quantities of bile salts have been found in the faeces from a cancer prone population compared with those from a low risk population.

A third hypothesis is that fat or protein in the diet is broken down into a potential carcinogen. There is also an association

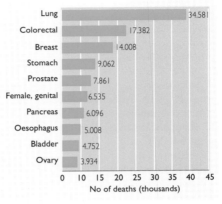

Fig 17.1 Deaths from cancers in England and Wales, 1989.

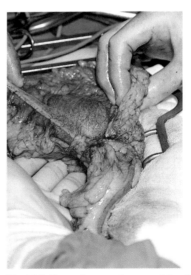

Fig 17.2 Stenosing carcinoma of the distal transverse colon.

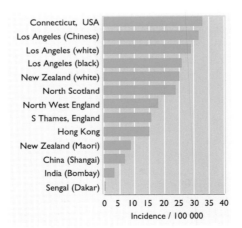

Fig 17.3 Global variation in colorectal cancer.

64

between smoking and alcohol consumption and colorectal neoplasia, but coffee drinking does not seem to be implicated.

Genetic factors

Family history—There is no doubt that some families have a high incidence of colorectal cancer. This is easily explained in those with familial adenomatous polyposis, which is inherited as an autosomal dominant condition. It accounts for only 1% of all colorectal cancers. Other families with a high incidence of large bowel cancer do not have familial adenomatous polyposis. Many of these have so called hereditary non-polyposis colon cancer (HNPCC), which is also inherited as an autosomal dominant condition and accounts for about 5% of patients with large bowel cancer. HNPCC kindreds are defined as those in which at least three relatives (one of whom is a first degree relative of the other two) are affected, with at least one diagnosed under the age of 50. The first degree relatives of patients who develop colorectal cancer before the age of 45, and those families in which multiple cancers occur, should also be considered as potential HNPCC kindreds.

Molecular biology—The recent revolution in molecular biology is uncovering a rapidly growing list of genetic abnormalities in patients with colorectal neoplasms. The most important genetic events are: (1) mutations that inactivate tumour suppressor genes and (2) mutations that activate oncogenes. In colorectal neoplasia these usually arise by point mutation or deletion of the relevant genes or segment of chromosome. These genetic events combine to influence tumour behaviour. Familial adenomatous polyposis arises due to a germ-line mutation of the adenomatous polyposis coli (APC) gene and HNPCC arises due to germ-line mutations in DNA mismatch repair genes (usually MSH2 or MHL1).

Predisposing diseases—Certain chronic diseases of the colon predispose to cancer. In particular, longstanding ulcerative colitis and, to a lesser extent, Crohn's disease are associated with carcinomatous change. Other causes of chronic inflammation, such as schistosomiasis, amoebic dysentery, and tuberculosis, do not seem to predispose to cancer. Implantation of the ureters into the sigmoid colon predisposes to large bowel neoplasia, but this form of urinary diversion has been largely abandoned. Cholecystectomy has been thought to be associated with an increased risk of colorectal cancer, but the evidence is equivocal.

Pathology

Large bowel cancers appear as polypoid, ulcerating, or stenosing lesions. They spread directly to invade local structures, this being especially important in rectal cancer owing to the proximity of the other pelvic structures. They metastasise through lymphatic vessels to mesenteric and para-aortic lymph nodes and through the portal venous system to the liver and onwards. Tumour cells may also be dispersed by transcoelomic spread across the abdominal cavity.

Colorectal cancers show a range of histological features, varying from well differentiated tumours with recognisable glandular structures to poorly differentiated lesions.

Patients may develop more than one large bowel carcinoma. The prevalence of multiplicity on presentation is variously quoted as between 3% and 12% of cases. These are so called synchronous tumours. There is also a higher incidence of further colorectal tumours after successful treatment of carcinoma of the colon. These are called metachronous tumours. Ten years after resection of a large bowel cancer there is a 3–4% incidence of a further malignancy in the remaining large bowel.

- A careful family history should be obtained from all patients with colorectal cancer
- Members of families with a significant history should be offered referral to a geneticist or interested specialist to assess their risk and need for screening

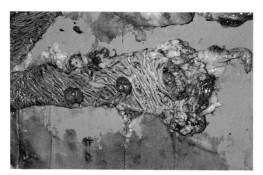
Fig 17.4 Pathological specimen showing familial adenomatous polyposis.

Conditions that predispose to large bowel cancer

- Ulcerative colitis
- Crohn's disease
- Familial adenomatous polyposis
- Hereditary non-polyposis colon cancer (HNPCC) (Lynch types I and II)
- Colonic ureteric implants
- Cholecystectomy (?)

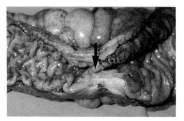
Fig 17.5 Pathological specimen showing stenosing colonic cancer.

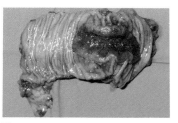
Fig 17.6 Ulcerating carcinoma.

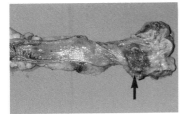

Fig 17.7 Rectal carcinoma close to the anus.

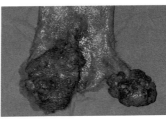

Fig 17.8 Coincident polyp and polypoid carcinoma.

Clinical features

The clinical features of colorectal cancer depend on the site of the tumour. About a quarter of large bowel tumours lie in the right side of the colon. The transverse and descending colon are relatively rarely affected so most lie in the sigmoid colon and rectum.

About a half of large bowel tumours are in the rectum. The clinical symptoms and signs differ depending on the area of bowel involved. From the point of view of symptoms it is best to consider three areas: the right colon, the left colon, and the rectum.

Right colon

Presentation with obstruction—About a quarter of the patients present with signs of low small bowel obstruction—that is, colic, vomiting, constipation, and distension. Plain abdominal radiographs show dilated loops of small bowel.

Presentation without obstruction—Many patients who present without obstruction have no symptoms referable to the gastrointestinal tract. They give a history of anaemia and weight loss as a result of occult gastrointestinal bleeding. This complex of symptoms raises the possibility of carcinoma of the stomach, but carcinoma of the right colon, which is much more amenable to treatment, is often overlooked. The diagnosis is suggested by the finding of a palpable mass in the right iliac fossa. Whether this is present or not the whole colon must be examined by colonoscopy or barium enema examination.

Left colon

Presentation with obstruction—In all, 25–30% of patients with lesions of the left colon present as an emergency. They may have a perforation with periocolic abscess or even general peritonitis, but more usually large bowel obstruction. By far the most common cause of large bowel obstruction is a carcinoma. It is important to exclude other causes of obstruction which may settle with conservative treatment. Emergency barium enema examination is indicated in all cases of large bowel obstruction to confirm the level of obstruction and to diagnose pseudo-obstruction, which does not require surgery. Emergency colonoscopy has been advocated as an alternative to barium enema examination.

Presentation without obstruction—Disturbance of the bowel habit is the rule in patients without obstruction. This may be either increasing constipation, diarrhoea, or alternation between the two. The patient commonly recognises blood with the stool and complains of low abdominal pain or discomfort. Weight loss is common and in general is a bad prognostic sign. A carcinoma can sometimes be felt by abdominal palpation.

Carcinoma of the rectum

Patients with carcinoma of the rectum almost never present as an emergency. The patient perceives obvious bleeding through the rectum. There may be alternation of the bowel habit and often tenesmus, a feeling of incomplete evacuation, with repeated calls to stool with the passage of only blood and slime. Tumours up to 10 cm from the anal verge can usually be

> **Two thirds of large bowel tumours lie in the rectum and sigmoid colon within reach of a flexible sigmoidoscope**

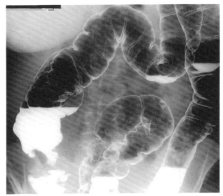

Fig 17.9 Barium enema radiograph showing carcinoma of the caecum.

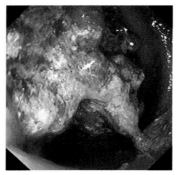

Fig 17.10 Endoscopic view of a carcinoma of the sigmoid colon.

felt. Tumours in the upper rectum can usually be seen on sigmoidoscopy.

Investigation

General abdominal, rectal, and sigmoidoscopic examination are part of the routine assessment of the patient in the clinic. If tumours are identified biopsy specimens are taken for histological confirmation. If no tumour is found on sigmoidoscopy either colonoscopy or barium enema examination should be performed. If a carcinoma is discovered synchronous tumours should be excluded. This may have to wait until the time of surgery or later if the tumour prevents adequate assessment of the more proximal colon. Ultrasonography and computed tomography may identify hepatic metastases, but their detection rarely precludes surgery as resection is largely the best form of palliation. Endoanal ultrasonography is emerging as a useful technique to assess the depth of penetration of rectal cancers, and may help stage and select patients for local excision or radiotherapy.

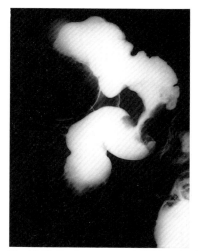

Fig 17.11 Barium enema radiograph of cancer of the sigmoid colon shows a characteristic "apple core" filling defect.

18 Colorectal neoplasia—III: Treatment and prevention

D J Jones

Carcinoma of the colon

The mainstay of treatment for large bowel cancer is still surgery with wide excision, including the appropriate lymph drainage areas. For most patients the appropriate excision would be a right or left hemicolectomy, but in some patients with several adenomas and young patients with cancer some surgeons advocate a total colectomy and ileorectal anastomosis. Radiotherapy has as yet played little part in the treatment of carcinoma of the colon.

Right colonic cancer

Cancer of the right colon with or without obstruction is treated by right hemicolectomy with primary anastomosis. Resection is indicated even in the presence of hepatic metastases because this gives the best palliation. In patients with manifest obstruction the operation has to be carried out as an emergency. Occasionally resection is not possible and the surgeon has to byass the tumour by anastomosing the ileum to the transverse colon.

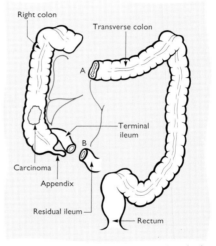

Fig 18.1 Bowel removal by right hemicolectomy. A is anastomosed to B.

Left colonic cancer

In the absence of intestinal obstruction the treatment of choice for cancer of the left colon is a wide excision by left hemicolectomy or sigmoid colectomy with primary anastomosis. Resection is carried out even in the presence of secondary tumours of the liver because this gives the best palliation. Colostomy alone is never justified in the absence of obstruction because it has little palliative value.

In cases of left colonic obstruction the traditional method was to use a three stage procedure: stage 1, colostomy alone; stage 2, resection with anastomosis; stage 3, closure of colostomy. In recent years there has been a tendency towards resection as the primary procedure. Often no anastomosis is attempted at the emergency operation. The upper residual colon is exteriorised as a colostomy and the lower colon is either exteriorised (by producing a mucus fistula) or closed (by Hartmann's procedure). A second operation can be carried out when the patient is fully recovered and intestinal continuity restored.

Some groups of surgeons go further and not only resect the tumour but also carry out primary anastomosis. This is helped by on table lavage of the colon, which clears faeces and reduces the disproportion in size between bowel above and below the resected carcinoma. A further option is to perform a subtotal colectomy and anastomose the small bowel to the distal residual colon or rectum. An ileorectal anastomosis should, however, be avoided in patients with a history of poor control or frank incontinence.

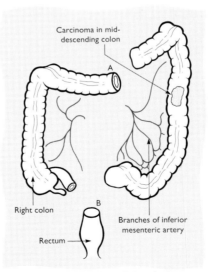

Fig 18.2 Procedure for left hemicolectomy. A is anastomosed to B.

Carcinoma of the rectum

Operable carcinoma of the upper half of the rectum can be adequately excised and anastomosis effected. This procedure is called anterior resection of the rectum. The anastomosis may be carried out by hand suture, but the advent of circular stapling devices has made it technically easier to carry out some low anterior resections.

The treatment options for cancers in the lower rectum are more varied. The standard treatment for tumours less than 6 cm from the anal margin is still abdominoperineal excision of the rectum (APER) with an end colostomy. Other treatment options have to be considered. Some tumours closer to the anus can be managed by rectal excision and coloanal anastomosis. Surgical technique is of great importance and local recurrence rates vary widely between different surgeons. Cancers rarely spread along the wall of the bowel, but involved lymph nodes may be found in the mesorectum up to 3 cm beyond the primary tumour. It is therefore recommended that the lymph node clearance should extend for 5 cm distal to the cancer. For cancers of the middle and lower thirds of the rectum, this necessitates a total mesorectal excision (TME) down to the pelvic floor with either a low rectal or coloanal anastomosis or an APER. The ability to perform a low anastomosis rather than an APER will be influenced by the patient's build and size of cancer. The short term functional results are improved if a colonic pouch is constructed in those requiring a coloanal anastomosis. Low rectal anastomoses are associated with an increased leak rate so the judicious use of a temporary covering colostomy or loop ileostomy is recommended in these patients.

Operative mortality and morbidity

In most centres the operative mortality rate for surgery in large bowel cancer is less than 5% and in some centres it is less than 2%. The operative mortality is higher if surgery is carried out for obstruction or perforation. The principal causes of death are coincident cardiorespiratory problems in elderly patients and leakage from an intestinal anastomosis. Anastomotic leakage varies in severity from a minor self limiting problem to a major life threatening one. Though there is a slight risk of leakage from any colonic anastomosis, the risk is greater in low colorectal anastomosis. The surgeon and the technique are the other associated factors in the incidence of anastomotic leakage.

Other non-fatal complications are wound infection and genitourinary dysfunction. Both the incidence and the severity of wound infection have been reduced by using perioperative antibiotics as prophylaxis against both aerobic and anaerobic organisms. Genitourinary dysfunction may manifest as either postoperative retention or later impotence. The principal cause of both of these is damage to the autonomic nerves within the pelvis.

Follow up programmes

The aim of any follow up programme should be to identify treatable recurrent disease as early as possible and to detect secondary metachronous carcinoma of the bowel. Regular clinical review is largely ineffective. For this reason attempts to detect asymptomatic recurrence or metachronous tumours are being assessed. Possible useful investigations may be endoscopy, assessment of tumour markers by blood sampling, and regular imaging by ultrasonography or computed tomography. Colonoscopy may lead to early detection of metachronous or recurrent tumours in asymptomatic patients. Measurement of carcinoembryonic antigen (CEA)

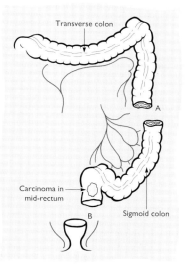

Fig 18.3 Procedure for anterior resection. A is anastomosed to B, restoring continuity.

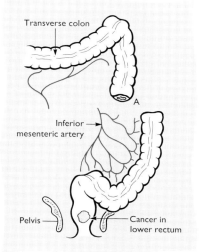

Fig 18.4 Procedure for abdominoperineal resection. A is exteriorised as an end colostomy.

Recommended treatment outcomes after surgery for colorectal cancer

Operative mortality <20% for emergency surgery

Operative mortality <5% for elective surgery
Anastomotic leak rate <8% after anterior resection
Anastomotic leak rate <4% for other anastomoses
Wound infection rate <10% after elective surgery
Local recurrence rate <10% after curative resection

Guidelines for the management of Colorectal Cancer.
The Royal College of Surgeons of England and the Association of Coloprocology of Great Britain and Ireland 1996

There is no evidence that intensive follow up to detect recurrent disease improves survival

It is reasonable to offer

- liver imaging to asymptomatic patients for the first two postoperative years to detect operable liver metastases
- colonoscopy every 3–5 years to detect metachronous cancers and polyps

concentration is the most usual test and if it becomes raised then intensive investigation with the potential of a "second look" laparotomy is considered. Unfortunately it is unusual to pick up recurrence amenable to curative resection.

Using ultrasonography or computed tomography to look for operable hepatic metastases is gaining acceptance. The frequency of scans and duration are uncertain, but most metastases are evident within two years of presentation. If the patient's general condition should preclude hepatic resection or chemotherapy, screening for metastatic disease would not be appropriate.

Recurrence

Most tumour recurrence becomes manifest in the first two years after surgery, though there is still a risk of recurrence after this time. Distant recurrence is most commonly seen in the liver. A solitary secondary deposit in the liver or lung may be the only evidence of recurrence. In this circumstance radical excision by partial hepatectomy or lobectomy is surprisingly effective. Local recurrence as a result of implantation of viable tumour cells at the anastomosis is rare. Local recurrence is usually caused by growth from extraluminal tumour deposits, which subsequently involve the bowel from without. For this reason a curative resection at "second look" laparotomy is rarely possible. Local recurrence is more common when the primary tumour was bulky, of high grade malignancy, or had associated lymph nodes, or if it was in the lower rectum.

Improving the results of surgery

The rate of local recurrence after rectal resection varies in different series from less than 5% to greater than 30%. This rate is related to the surgeon and the extent of local spread. Even radical resection may be incomplete because lymphatic chains extend beyond the limits of resection. Rectal cancer may recur in the lymphatic tissue of the lateral pelvic wall.

A margin of 2 cm distal to the tumour is considered adequate to remove radically all intramural tumour, but the mesorectum requires special attention. Inadequate removal of the mesorectum leaves potentially affected lymph nodes. Careful meticulous attention to dissection of the mesorectum is believed to reduce local recurrence rates.

Radiotherapy

Radiotherapy given either before or after the operation decreases the rate of local recurrence of rectal cancers. If given before the operation the tumour is easily targeted and it does not increase the risks of subsequent surgery. A minority of patients will be found to have early disease; radiotherapy does not confer any additional benefit for these patients. Patients can be selected for postoperative radiotherapy on the basis of the operative and pathological findings, but small bowel may lie in the radiotherapy field in the pelvis and is at risk of significant radiation injury. Although radiotherapy reduces the rate of local recurrence it does not seem to prolong survival as patients die of distant metastases outside the radiotherapy field.

Chemotherapy
Adjuvant therapy

At present there is no clear indication for routine adjuvant chemotherapy outside of clinical trials. Although individual studies show no benefit, meta-analysis of published randomised trials has shown a slight survival advantage for patients treated with 5-fluorouracil. A US study has suggested some improved survival for patients given a combination of 5-fluorouracil and

Age corrected survival of survivors of curative resection	82%	(99/121)
Age corrected survival after curative resection	77%	(99/128)
Crude survival after curative resection	70%	(89/128)
Crude tumour free survival after curative resection	63%	(81/128)
Crude survival	47%	(89/189)
Crude tumour free survival of referred patients	43%	(81/189)
Age corrected survival of survivors of histological curative resection	89%	(93/104)
Age corrected survival after histological curative resection	85%	(93/110)
Crude survival after histological curative resection	76%	(84/110)

Fig 18.5 Different ways of reporting survival in a group of 189 patients. Survival at three years varies from 43% to 89% depending on the criteria adopted.

Types of recurrence
- Local
- Distant
  —Liver only
  —Lung only
  —Diffuse

Radiotherapy in the treatment of rectal cancer
- Short term high dose pre-operative radiotherapy should be considered for all patients with clinically operable rectal cancer.
- Short term high dose pre-operative radiotherapy is indicated where the surgeon is not confident of achieving a histologically curative resection.
- Patients with fixed rectal cancers should be considered for a long course of radiotherapy followed by further assessment of operability and attempted resection if feasible.
- Patients with involved circumferential margins after surgery without pre-operative radiotherapy should be considered for post-operative radiotherapy

---

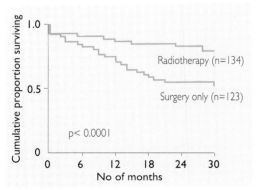

Fig 18.6 Local recurrence free survival in those receiving surgery only and in those receiving preoperative radiotherapy in a randomised controlled trial.

levamisole. The action of fluorouracil is potentiated by folinic acid. The role of these agents is under further evaluation in the QUASAR trial. Adjuvant intraportal 5-fluorouracil given through a catheter introduced at laparotomy has been under investigation in the United Kingdom in the AXIS trial (Adjuvant X-ray and Infusion Study).

Advanced disease

5-Fluorouracil is also the best drug for patients with advanced disease, but the response rate is poor and toxicity of treatment may impair the quality of life. Hepatic artery infusion of 5-fluorouracil with or without chemoembolisation with degradable starch microspheres may reduce systemic toxicity and is under evaluation.

> Patients with Dukes' stage C colorectal cancer (involved lymph nodes) should be offered entry into a trial or considered for fluorouracil containing adjuvant chemotherapy

---

> **UK chemotherapy trials for advanced diseases**
>
> **CR05** Patients with advanced colorectal cancer confined to the liver are randomised to receive either systemic intravenous 5-fluorouracil or intra-hepatic arterial 5-flourouracil and leucovorin.
>
> **CR06** Patients with advanced colorectal cancer randomised to compare three systemic chemotherapy regimes.

Prognosis

The life expectancy of a patient with large bowel cancer depends on the degree of spread at presentation. Factors which adversely affect the prognosis are distant metastases, local spread causing fixation to irremovable structures, high histological grade malignancy, and spread to regional lymph nodes. For all patients outcome in terms of survival is about 25%, but in patients thought to have a curable resection at operation it is better than 50%, and if the tumour has not penetrated the full thickness of the colonic wall there is almost normal life expectancy.

There are many different methods of staging large bowel cancer; most use an ABC classification introduced by Dukes. They are not directly comparable and the prefix "Dukes" is often used erroneously.

Histological involvement of the lateral resection margin of a rectal cancer specimen is an important predictor of local recurrence. Cancers extending to within 1 mm of a circumferential margin should be considered as incompletely resected and deemed non-curative even if all macroscopic tumour was thought to have been excised.

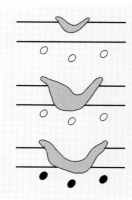

A Confined to the bowel wall. Excellent long term prognosis after curative resection

B Spread through the bowel wall. A half to two-thirds become long term survivors after curative resection

C Lymph node metastases. Most but not all will have spread through the bowel wall. Poor prognosis. Only a quarter become long term survivors after curative resection

Fig 18.7 Dukes' staging. This form is probably the most popular in the United Kingdom.

Prevention

Population screening

Randomised Controlled Trials in the United States of America, Denmark, and the United Kingdom have shown that screening average risk individuals may help reduce mortality from colorectal cancer, although the tests have considerable limitations. The method is to test for blood in the faeces and to investigate subjects with positive test results. There are several simple tests, usually based on guaiac impregnated stips which change colour in the presence of blood (Haemoccult, Faecotest). One dilemma of occult blood testing is that if the test is very sensitive it yields huge numbers of false positive results, whereas if it is of low sensitivity false negative results occur.

All studies have had difficulty in getting good patient acceptance of screening procedures. Investigation of patients with positive test results should include clinical examination and colonoscopy. Most studies have shown a good yield of minor colonic disturbances but only a modest number of carcinomas. In some studies the cancers diagnosed appear to be at an earlier pathological stage.

The cost for a national screening using faecal occult blood tests would demand a substantial commitment of resources, and such a programme has not yet been established.

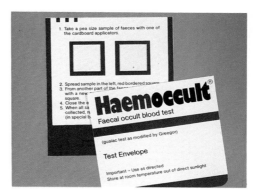

Fig 18.8 Haemoccult test card. A sample of faeces is smeared on the test card. Hydrogen peroxide is added in the laboratory. A blue colour changes indicates the presence of blood.

Endoscopic screening is probably more effective and two thirds of cases of large bowel cancer are within reach of the facilities of a flexible sigmoidoscopy. In the United Kingdom a multicentre study (Flexiscope trial) evaluating the role of screening by flexible sigmoidoscopy has started. If shown to be effective population screening would demand a substantial commitment of resources.

Individual screening

Some people are known to have a high risk of developing large bowel cancer. Screening of people from families with a history of cancer, polyposis, and inflammatory bowel disease is now generally accepted. Any adenomas detected are removed and patients with multiple adenomas are treated by prophylactic excisional surgery.

Causes of positive result on testing for faecal occult blood

- Hiatus hernia
- Peptic ulcer
- Piles and other minor anal disease
- Colonic adenoma
- Carcinoma of the colon

High risk groups

- People with a family history of familial polyposis
- People with a strong family history of large bowel cancer (HNPCC kindreds)
- People with longstanding ulcerative colitis
- People who have undergone resection of colonic carcinoma or a polyp

---

Useful organisations

BACUP (British Association of Cancer United Patients)
3 Bath Place
Rivington Street
London EC2A 3JR

British Colostomy Association
15 Station Road
Reading
Berkshire RG1 1LG

19 Anal cancer

R D James, S T O'Dwyer

Anal cancer is relatively uncommon, accounting for about 4% of anorectal malignancies. The condition is of increasing interest owing to appreciable changes in the patterns of treatment. The traditional treatment for anal cancer was a radical abdominoperineal excision, leaving the patient with a permanent colostomy. Emerging evidence shows that most anal cancers respond to a combination of radiotherapy and chemotherapy, which improves survival and enables radical surgery to be avoided.

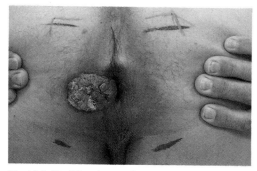

Fig 19.1 Proliferative anal cancer.

Pathology

About 80% of anal malignancies are squamous cell carcinomas. They show a range of histological features, varying from predominantly well differentiated keratinising large cell tumours at the anal margin to less differentiated non-keratinising small cell carcinomas in the upper anal canal. The precise histological pattern is rarely important, but their position in the anus influences clinical decisions.

Anal canal carcinomas arise at or above the dentate line and are not visible at the anus.

Anal margin cancers occur below the dentate line and are visible; they behave like basal cell skin carcinomas and have a more favourable prognosis than anal canal cancers. If advanced the position of origin is difficult to determine.

Anal carcinomas appear as ulcers or proliferative growths with ulcerated areas. They become hard and fixed as the malignancy progresses. They spread directly to invade the underlying anal sphincters, which are affected in three quarters of patients at presentation. Tumours above the dentate line spread to the superior haemorrhoidal lymph nodes while those below the dentate line metastasise to the inguinal lymph nodes.

Types of anal neoplasm
- Squamous cell carcinoma
- Malignant melanoma
- Lymphoma
- Anal gland adenocarcinoma

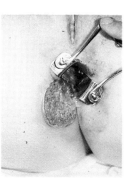

Fig 19.2 Ulcerating cancer of the anal margin.

Aetiology

There is an increased incidence of anal cancer among male homosexuals, people who practise anal intercourse, and those with a history of genital warts. This knowledge prompted a search for a sexually transmitted agent which may be implicated in the pathogenesis of anal cancer. A corollary has been drawn with cervical cancer and its association with human papillomavirus infection. A half of patients with anal cancer have human papillomavirus types 16 and 18 DNA incorporated in the genome of their tumour cells. Some patients with genital warts have evidence of intraepithelial neoplasia around the anus, analogous to cervical intraepithelial neoplasia, which is recognised to be a premalignant condition. Though some of this evidence may be circumstantial, there is growing concern that the increasing incidence of genital human papillomavirus infection will ultimately lead to an increased incidence of anal cancer.

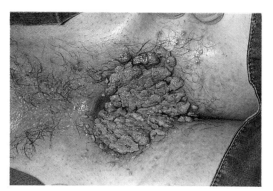

Fig 19.3 Perianal papillomas are increasing in incidence and may predispose to anal cancer.

Clinical features

Overall anal cancers are more common in women, although lesions at the anal margin are more common in men. Most patients are in their 50s or 60s. They present with bleeding, pain, swelling, and ulceration around the anus. As the tumour advances patients suffer worsening pain, disturbed bowel habit, incontinence, and rectovaginal fistulas. Many patients have enlarged inguinal lymph nodes, but only 50% of paplable glands contain tumour.

Early cancers may be confused with papillomas, warts, fissures, and haemorrhoids, which may lead to delay in diagnosis and treatment. Clinical examination under anaesthesia is usually necessary as local tenderness often prevents thorough assessment. Local spread into surrounding structures is determined and biopsy specimens taken for histological confirmation and classification.

Treatment

The traditional treatment for anal cancer was a radical abdominoperineal resection and a permanent colostomy. In 1974 an American report suggested that patients with anal cancer could be cured by a combination of 5-fluorouracil and mitomycin. At the same time there were reports from France and the United Kingdom on the curative effects of radiotherapy. Within a few years primary surgical treatment was replaced by radiotherapy with concomitant chemotherapy.

A recent British trial randomised 577 eligible patients to receive either radiotherapy or chemotherapy in addition to 5-fluorouracil with mitomycin C. There was a 54% reduction in the risk of local treatment failure and a reduced risk of death from anal cancer in patients receiving combined modality treatment. The addition of chemotherapy to radiotherapy did not add appreciably to either early or late treatment co-morbidity. Co-trimoxazole prophylaxis was used in the combined mortality arm to reduce the risk of infection. A recent RTOG/ELOG intergroup trial showed statistically significant advantage in terms of local failure, colostomy, and disease free survival for 5-fluorouracil + mitomycin + radiotherapy when compared with 5-fluorouracil + radiotherapy.

All patients with anal cancer should be assessed jointly by a radiotherapist and a surgeon. The vast majority should be offered radical radiotherapy with 5-fluorouracil and mitomycin chemotherapy, with surgery held in reserve for cases in which this fails. All patients should preferably be entered into a clinical trial because this is a comparatively rare tumour.

The initial radiotherapy field includes the tumour and the inguinal lymph nodes. The patient is treated over 4–5 weeks. This inevitably gives rise to moist desquamation of the perineum. Young women should be warned that they will suffer an artificial menopause and men will be azoospermic. The skin heals three weeks after the completion of radiotherapy. A boost is generally given to the primary tumour by using a radioisotope. This requires a short general anaesthetic.

All cytotoxic agents carry a measurable risk. There is an argument for omitting cytotoxic agents in good risk patients, mainly those with T1 tumours. They should be used with caution in elderly people. Their main risk is thrombocytopenia and agranulocytosis caused by mitomycin, and most oncologists prescribe antibiotic prophylaxis (co-trimoxazole). 5-Fluorouracil, which has a very short biological half life, must be given by slow infusion to ensure synergy with radiation.

Staging of anal cancers

Anal canal modified (Papillon, 1982)

T1	<2 cm
T2	2–5 cm
T3	>5 cm
T4a	Invading vaginal mucosa
T4b	Invading surrounding structures other than skin, rectum, or vagina
Tx	Insufficient information available

Anal margin

T1	<2 cm
T2	2–5 cm
T3	>5 cm
T4	Extension to muscle, bone, etc

Combined treatment arm of the United Kingdom anal cancer trial

4500 cGy in 20/25 fractions in 4/5 weeks plus boost *and*
5-Fluorouracil 1000 mg/m^2/24 hours on days 1–4
Mitomycin C 12 mg/m^2 on day 1 only
Repeat treatment with 5-fluorouracil in final week of radiotherapy

---

Fig 19.4 Desquamation of the perineum caused by initial radiotherapy field. This patient's skin was completely healed three weeks later.

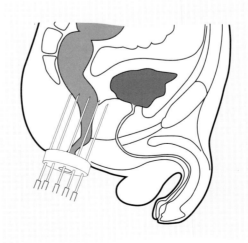

Fig 19.5 Device for administering boost radiotherapy treatment.

The rate of cure for combined modality radiotherapy and chemotherapy is about 60%, but many failures of treatment of local tumours can be salvaged by abdominoperineal resection. Aggressive tumours metastasise to the liver and occasionally to the bones, abdominal lymph nodes, or even the brain. Chemotherapy in these patients can often produce a remission of several months.

Surgery

Radical surgery is now reserved for patients who fail to respond to chemoradiation and patients with obstructive cancers who benefit from a colostomy while they undergo treatment. Surgery is also indicated for small cancers at the anal margin which are less than 2 cm in diameter and have not invaded the anal sphincter. They can be excised locally, but less than 5% of anal cancers fulfil these criteria.

Prognosis

For prognostic purposes most information of clinical value is obtained by distinguishing tumours arising at the anal margin from those in the anal canal and separating them into those greater or less than 5 cm in diameter. The tumour is relatively uncommon so there have been relatively few large follow up studies, but the five year survival rate is about 50%.

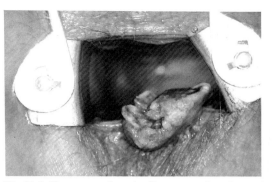

Fig 19.6 Tumours <5 cm in diameter and at the anal margin have a more favourable prognosis.

The photographs were prepared by the department of medical illustration, Christie Hospital and Holt Radium Institute. The full anal UKCCR trial protocol is available from the CRC Clinical Trial Centre, Rayne Institute, London.

20 Intestinal stomas

S Hughes, M H Irving

A stoma is a surgically created opening of the bowel or urinary tract on to the body surface. The most common procedures for producing intestinal stomas are ileostomy, colostomy, and urostomy.

Types of stoma

There are several different types of stoma.

End stomas—These are the simplest to create. The divided bowel is brought through the abdominal wall and anastomosed to the skin.

Loop stomas—These are created when a mobile loop of bowel—of necessity either the small bowel or the mobile parts of the colon (transverse or sigmoid)—is brought through the abdominal wall and the margins sewn to the skin. Loop stomas are usually temporary, being used to protect anastomoses distal to the stoma or divert bowel contents away from diseased segments further down the bowel such as an obstructing lesion or multiple perineal fistulas. Such stomas are prone to complications and because of their bulk are difficult to manage.

Continent stomas—These are those in which surgical techniques are used to create a valve like mechanism in the bowel proximal to the cutaneous opening which will allow discharge of faecal contents only when intubated. When successful, such a valve avoids the need for a patient to wear an appliance.

Other ways of creating openings on the abdominal wall include caecostomy, by which the caecum is intubated with a Foley catheter, which is commonly inserted through the stump of the removed appendix. Flatus and liquid faeces can escape through the lumen of the catheter.

The distal end of a divided segment of bowel can be closed and returned to the abdomen as in the Hartmann's procedure, but it is often brought to the abdominal surface and sutured to the skin and is then termed a "mucus fistula".

Stoma care nurses

Although the patient's doctor will be the first to suggest that a stoma will be necessary, preoperative explanation and counselling will usually be undertaken by a stoma care nurse, who is specially trained in the management of patients with all types of stomas. A certificate in Stoma Care Nursing (ENB 216) is now incorporated within a diploma/degree programme at two new centres within the United Kingdom. Other minor courses are available in the country.

Siting the stoma

The presence of a stoma is enough of a burden for a patient, and the burden is increased enormously if the stoma is badly sited or badly constructed. To avoid the problem of bad siting the stoma care nurse should examine the patient before operation to determine the ideal position.

Features to be taken into account are the nature of the skin surrounding the proposed stoma—ideally it should be flat and

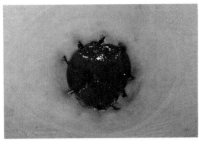

Fig 20.1 End stoma.

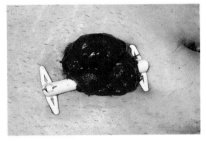

Fig 20.2 Loop stoma.

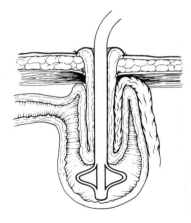

Fig 20.3 Continent stoma with catheter in pouch.

ENB 216 courses
- Hope Hospital, Salford
- St Bartholomew's Hospital, London

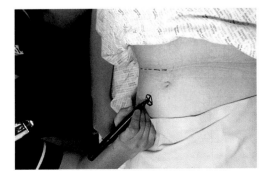

Fig 20.4 Stoma care nurse siting a stoma.

free from scars—and the presence of anatomical irregularities such as the umbilicus and anterior superior iliac spine. Note should also be taken of clothing, such as the position of belts.

Construction of the stoma

It is not only the site of stoma that is important but also its shape. Badly constructed stomas are difficult to control and rapidly lead to deterioration in morale. The two most common stomas are the ileal and colostomy stomas.

The end ileostomy, usually situated in the right iliac fossa, is normally constructed after panproctocolectomy for colitis. It discharges liquid faeces, which will excoriate and digest unprotected skin. For this reason the ideal ileostomy has a short spout created by everting the divided ileum back on itself. This spout ensures that the faeces can be projected into the lumen of the stoma bag.

The end colostomy usually discharges solid faeces intermittently. Although still capable of causing contact dermatitis on the surrounding skin, the faeces are not as corrosive. Because of this the stoma formed from the sigmoid colon can be flush with the skin, the solid faeces falling into the stoma bag.

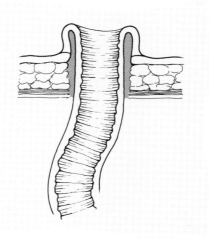

Fig 20.5 Ileostomy showing eversion to produce a spout.

Management

Appliances

The key to successful management of a stoma is a well constructed and well fitting appliance. There are many different types of appliance, though all work on the same principle.

The base is a sheet of adhesive with a hole which can be adjusted by the patient to fit the stoma. Irregularities and discrepancies can be filled in with pastes. On to the sheet of adhesive is fixed a ring of plastic or other material, from which the bag originates. The bag itself is made of thin flexible plastic and may be vented to allow the escape of gas. The lower end of the bag may have a removable seal to allow emptying of faeces. Alternatively a full bag may be removed and thrown away.

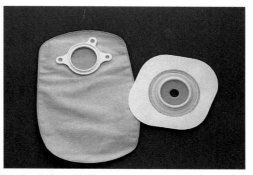

Fig 20.6 Base plate (right) is applied to skin around stoma with a clip on the bag.

Sophisticated management

Many patients seek to disguise the presence of a stoma or to avoid wearing a bag. Special clothing such as special swimwear is available.

Colonic stomas can be washed out by irrigating them, which, if successful, means the patient need not wear a bag.

Various occlusive devices have been developed to try to contain the faecal discharge until it is convenient to evacuate it. However, with rare exception, they have not proved effective and few patients use them.

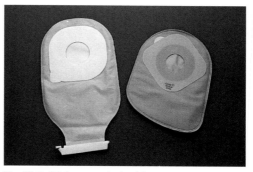

Fig 20.7 Right: non-drainable stoma bag. Left: drainable stoma bag which can be emptied without removing bag.

Complications

Many problems can arise with both the structure and function of stomas. Diarrhoea and constipation can usually be controlled by drugs, but anatomical defects often need surgical correction.

Prolapse of a stoma looks alarming and is unsightly and uncomfortable but rarely is dangerous. It can be corrected by surgery.

Stenosis causes obstruction of the faecal discharge and if untreated can be serious. Local dilatation is tempting but rarely successful; it should be treated by refashioning the stoma.

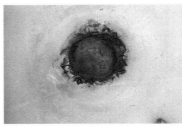

Fig 20.8 Necrotic ileostomy 48 hours after surgery. The necrotic mucosa eventually sloughed, leaving a healthy ileostomy.

Skin rashes are usually the result of failure of an appliance to fit snugly around the stoma. Occasionally they result from contact dermatitis caused by the components of the stoma bag.

Parastomal hernia is a common problem, especially in patients who have had a colostomy. If mild it does not require any treatment. If troublesome it can commonly be controlled by a supporting belt. If severe it can be repaired by surgery.

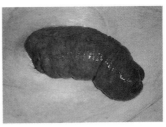
Fig 20.9 Prolapsed stoma.

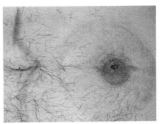
Fig 20.10 Stenosed stoma.

Patient welfare

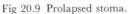

> **Voluntary organisations**
> - British Colostomy Association,
>   15 Station Road,
>   Reading,
>   Berkshire
> - Ileostomy Association,
>   Amblehurst Lane,
>   Black Scotch Lane,
>   Mansfield,
>   Nottinghamshire NG18 4PF

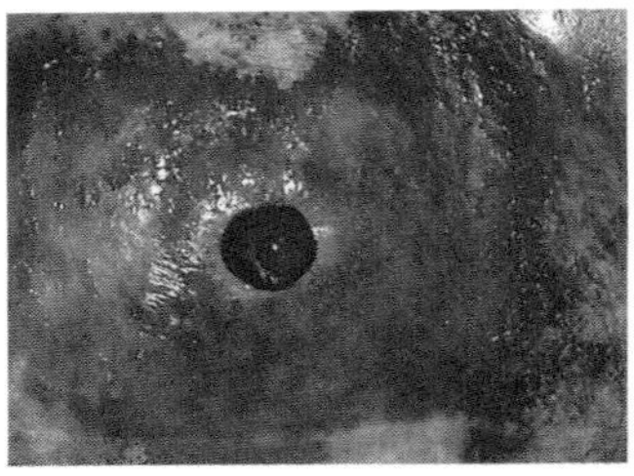

Most patients cope well with their stoma. They may benefit from association, however, with one of the voluntary organisations for the welfare of patients with stomas.

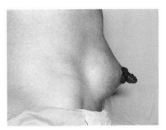
Fig 20.11 Peristomal rash.

Fig 20.12 Parastomal hernia.

21   Large bowel volvulus

D J Jones

In volvulus the colon twists on its own mesenteric axis, causing partial or complete obstruction of the large bowel. The blood supply of the colon is compromised because of venous congestion, which occasionally progresses to venous infarction and gangrene. Less commonly the arterial supply is compromised, leading to more rapid colonic ischaemia.

The most common site for large bowel volvulus is the sigmoid colon, which twists in an anticlockwise direction. The caecum is affected less commonly and twists in a clockwise direction; the transverse colon rarely undergoes volvulus. Occasionally a loop of ileum may become trapped within the volvulus, causing concomitant small bowel obstruction.

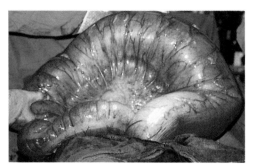

Fig 21.1 Sigmoid volvulus.

Sigmoid volvulus

Sigmoid volvulus accounts for about 5% of cases of large bowel obstruction in developed countries. It occurs predominantly in elderly people, with an increased incidence in patients with chronic medical and psychiatric disorders. Volvulus is more common in Africa and Asia, where it is the most common cause of large bowel obstruction. It is postulated that both a high fibre diet and chronic constipation may stretch the colon, leading to a long, narrow based sigmoid mesentery, which predisposes to volvulus.

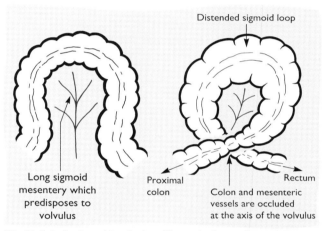

Fig 21.2 Left: sigmoid volvulus. The twist is usually anticlockwise. Right: sigmoid colon after volvulus

Clinical features

Patients with sigmoid volvulus present with colicky abdominal pain, constipation, failure to pass flatus, nausea, and vomiting. They have appreciable abdominal distension, which is usually much greater than that seen in patients with large bowel obstruction caused by a tumour. The distension may be sufficient to affect cardiac and respiratory function. The rectum tends to be ballooned and devoid of faeces.

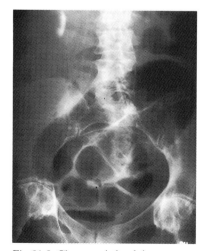

Fig 21.3 Characteristic plain abdominal radiograph showing distended sigmoid colon.

Diagnosis

In most patients the diagnosis is suspected on the basis of clinical features and the characteristic grossly dilated sigmoid loop on supine abdominal radiography. Sigmoidoscopy and colonoscopy provide an opportunity both to confirm the diagnosis and to decompress the obstructed loop. A single contrast barium enema examination is occasionally necessary to differentiate volvulus from pseudo-obstruction and obstruction caused by a tumour.

Treatment

Sigmoidoscopy should be performed, and this can be done at the bedside. The narrowing is usually less than 25 cm from the anal margin, within reach of a standard rigid sigmoidoscope. The instrument itself will occasionally pass into the obstructed segment, but it is usually necessary to introduce a well lubricated rectal or flatus tube. When successful there is a sudden, often dramatic release of liquid faeces and flatus. The tube can be left in place to prevent early relapse but is usually removed on decompression for the patient's comfort. If rigid sigmoidoscopy is unsuccessful the distended loop can often be decompressed by using a colonoscope or flexible sigmoidoscope.

About half of patients in whom decompression is successful will suffer further episodes of volvulus within two years. If the patient's general condition permits, early elective sigmoid colectomy after bowel preparation is the treatment of choice. Urgent laparotomy is indicated if the bowel cannot be decompressed or if the released contents are blood stained, suggesting colonic necrosis.

Surgery

Patients undergoing surgery for volvulus should have their legs raised and extended in supports to permit access to the anus. The abdomen is opened and the colon untwisted. The bowel can then be decompressed by introducing a flatus tube through the anus, which the abdominal surgeon manipulates into the distended loop.

Most patients are suitable for sigmoid colectomy and primary anastomosis. If the bowel is loaded with faeces, an on table irrigation of the colon may be performed. If there is doubt about the viability of the colon or there is appreciable intra-abdominal sepsis, a primary anastomosis should not be performed. The proximal colon is exteriorised as an end colostomy and the rectal stump oversewn (Hartmann's procedure). An alternative is to exteriorise the proximal and distal colon side by side as a double barrelled colostomy (the Paul–Mickulicz procedure). When the patient has recovered, the common wall can be crushed with an enterotome, or nowadays more easily divided by using a linear stapler cutter. Faeces can then pass into the distal colon, allowing the stoma to close spontaneously. Common problems with the double barrelled colostomy were necrosis of the distal limb and failure of closure of the colostomy, and this procedure is no longer the preferred option. A sigmoidopexy, fixing the colon to the abdominal wall, seems an attractive option to prevent recurrent volvulus; however, it is usually ineffective and should be avoided.

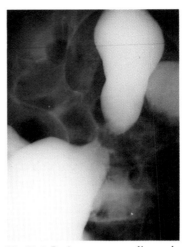

Fig 21.4 Barium enema radiograph showing characteristic tapered occlusion of the sigmoid colon as a result of volvulus.

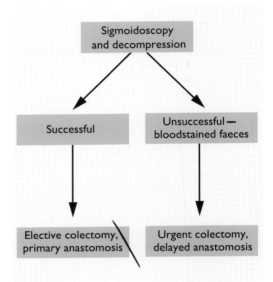

Fig 21.5 Management of large bowel volvulus.

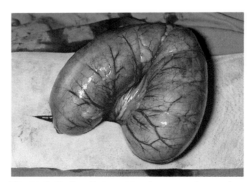

Fig 21.6 Deflated sigmoid volvulus before elective resection.

Caecal volvulus

Caecal volvulus is less common than sigmoid volvulus, and patients usually present with a short history and have symptoms and signs of acute intestinal obstruction. Characteristic radiological patterns may be observed, but the precise cause of obstruction is rarely distinguished preoperatively.

At laparotomy the bowel is untwisted. The preferred option is to perform a right hemicolectomy with primary ileocolic anastomosis. An alternative is simply to insert a caecostomy tube after untwisting the caecum. This serves to fix the caecum to the abdominal wall and prevent further episodes of volvulus. Recurrent volvulus is, however, more likely than after resection, and emergency right hemicolectomy is a safe procedure.

Pseudo-obstruction

Pseudo-obstruction is characterised by pronounced abdominal distension suggestive of large bowel obstruction in the absence of an obstructing lesion. It is important to recognise the condition in order to avoid unnecessary surgery. It often arises in patients with other medical conditions and in patients in hospital. The distension is impressive but there is usually minimal pain and vomiting. Abdominal radiographs show colonic distension which may be segmental.

Occasionally caecal distension may be sufficient to threaten perforation, but the distension can usually be relieved by sigmoidoscopy or colonoscopy, which may need to be repeated. An instant barium enema examination will exclude a mechanical lesion.

Surgery is not the treatment of choice for pseudo-obstruction and carries a high morbidity and mortality in frail, elderly patients. It is indicated only on the rare occasions when the clinical signs suggest that caecal perforation is likely.

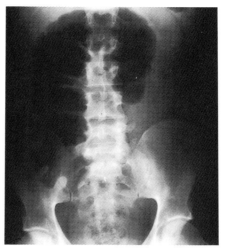

Fig 21.7 Plain abdominal radiograph showing dilated caecum secondary to volvulus.

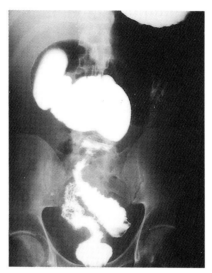

Fig 21.8 Barium enema examination was performed to exclude a mechanical obstruction in a patient with pseudo-obstruction. Barium enema examination or colonoscopy should be performed in all patients with suspected large bowel obstuction to avoid unnecessary surgery in those with pseudo-obstruction.

22 Colorectal trauma

D J Jones

Trauma of the large bowel is relatively uncommon in the United Kingdom. Colorectal injury occurs after blunt or penetrating trauma and the introduction of foreign bodies into the rectum.

Major abdominal trauma

Blunt abdominal trauma—That caused by road traffic accidents is the most common type of injury in the United Kingdom; patients usually have multiple injuries. Bowel injury arises from direct impact and deceleration, which cause shearing and rotational forces, culminating in burst bowel and torn mesentery. Seat belt injury is the classic form. The colon is injured in less than 5% of patients with major blunt abdominal trauma, and injuries to the liver, spleen, kidneys, and small bowel are far more common.

Penetrating trauma—In the United Kingdom this is usually the result of stabbings and less commonly of low velocity firearms. The incidence of stab wounds is increasing, especially in inner cities. Abdominal viscera are at risk of injury with any penetrating wound below the nipples. The large bowel is injured in about 10% of abdominal stabbings, the transverse colon being the most vulnerable segment. More serious penetrating injuries are inflicted by high velocity weapons and debris from bomb blasts. Visceral injury is present in three quarters of those with gunshot injuries. Soldiers are at risk of rectal injury from gunshot wounds sustained while lying on the ground in the characteristic prone position.

Injury resulting from the introduction of objects into the rectum for self gratification is also becoming more common. Most patients present because they are no longer able to remove the object. Serious associated injury to the bowel is uncommon.

Management

The resuscitation and management of a patient with major abdominal trauma follows the established sequence for all victims of major trauma. A primary survey is performed and the patient resuscitated. A secondary survey identifies all the injuries and definitive management is initiated.

A history of the incident is obtained from the patient or witnesses to determine the mechanism of injury which gives clues to the likely injuries. The abdomen is notoriously difficult to assess by clinical examination. Muscle guarding and signs of peritoneal irritation are commonly present in the multiply injured patient and their importance may be uncertain. Bowel sounds are unhelpful as their presence or absence does not help determine whether or not there is a significant injury.

Unequivocal evidence of major intra-abdominal injury is an indication for surgical intervention. A diagnostic peritoneal lavage is performed if abdominal examination is equivocal, unreliable, or impractical and in patients with unexplained hypotension. This shows evidence of major intra-abdominal haemorrhage and ruptured viscera. A rectal examination is performed to detect blood, loss of integrity of the bowel wall, and a high lying prostate.

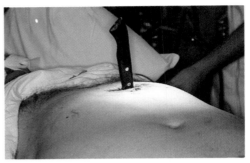

Fig 22.1 Penetrating weapons should not be removed before operation.

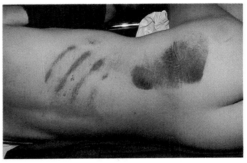

Fig 22.2 Bruising over the ribs after blunt abdominal trauma; there is a high risk of major thoracic and intra-abdominal injury.

Initial assessment and resuscitation of patients with major trauma

- Primary survey and resuscitation
  Airway and cervical spine control
  Breathing
  Circulation and haemorrhage control
  Dysfunction of the central nervous system
  Exposure
- Secondary survey
- Definitive management

Information required about the incident

- Medical history of patient
- Nature of incident:
  Stabbing
  Shooting
- In road traffic accidents:
  Speed of vehicle
  Nature of impact
  Deformation of vehicle
  Steering wheel involvement
  Seat belt involvement
- Injuries to other victims

Investigations

In patients with major injuries blood is taken for cross matching and to determine the haemoglobin concentration, white cell count, and urea and electrolyte concentrations. Radiographs of the chest and pelvis are taken. Computed tomography and ultrasonography, if available, are useful in the assessment of the stable patient who does not require an immediate laparotomy. Specific injuries to the large bowel, however, are rarely identified by preoperative investigations.

Diagnostic peritoneal lavage may still be needed after computed tomography or ultrasonography because these do not distinguish between blood and bowel contents, which would indicate visceral perforation.

Large bowel injury

Management

Stab wounds—At one stage it was customary to explore all abdominal stab wounds. An expectant policy with active observation is now preferred in patients who do not have signs of major intra-abdominal haemorrhage or peritonitis. Laparotomy is performed if the patient develops signs of such injury.

Firearm wounds—All patients with gunshot wounds which may have involved the abdomen should undergo laparotomy.

Blunt injury—If there is evidence of major intra-abdominal haemorrhage, peritonism suggestive of a ruptured viscus, or a peritoneal lavage proves positive, a laparotomy is performed. If there is not an immediate indication for laparotomy a policy of active observation is adopted and surgery performed if injuries become apparent.

The management of the large bowel injury itself is controversial. Debate centres around the relative merits of débridement, repair, and exteriorisation of bowel ends versus primary repair or resection and primary anastomosis. During the two World Wars mortality from colorectal trauma, particularly in those treated by primary closure, was so high (60%) that the surgeon general of the US Army issued an order requiring all large bowel injuries to be treated by colostomy. This policy was followed in Korea and Vietnam with a dramatic reduction in mortality as a result of colorectal trauma. Such a rigid policy is not considered necessary in civilian practice, where victims receive prompt medical attention. The risks of sepsis are lower and selected injuries can be treated by primary repair or resection with anastomosis.

Types of injury

Injury to the large bowel results in three types of injury: simple tears; mesenteric injuries which bleed and devascularise the bowel; and complex injuries with major disruption of both bowel and mesentery. If bowel contents are released into the peritoneal cavity, faecal peritonitis soon develops.

Simple tears—These tears of the bowel can be safely repaired without the aid of a proximal defunctioning colostomy.

Mesentric tears—These tears require sutures and ligatures to control haemorrhage. If there is doubt about the viability of the bowel it should be resected.The proximal colon is exteriorised as an end colostomy and the distal bowel either exteriorised as a mucus fistula if there is sufficient length or, alternatively, oversewn. In selected cases a primary anastomosis may be performed.

Complex injuries—Such injuries to the left colon usually necessitate resection and exteriorisation of the bowel end. In

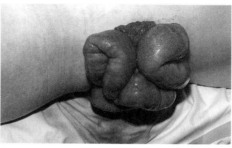
Fig 22.3 Visceral prolapse after stab wound in the left loin.

Indications for laparotomy

- Unexplained hypotension
- Evisceration
- Pneumoperitoneum on radiography
- Gunshot wounds
- Positive results on peritoneal lavage
- Definite signs of bleeding
- Definite signs of visceral rupture

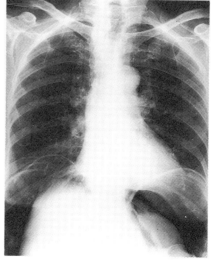
Fig 22.4 Radiograph showing pneumoperitonium after perforation of the colon during colonoscopy.

the absence of extreme faecal contamination and other major injuries, primary anastomosis is becoming increasingly more appropriate. If the injury affected the rectum the presacral space should be drained.

Large bowel injuries carry a high risk of clostridial sepsis, so appropriate antibiotics should be given. Bowel continuity is restored and colostomies are closed at a later date when the patient has recovered.

Primary repair

About half of all large bowel injuries are suitable for primary repair or resection and anastomosis. This line of management is, however, contraindicated in the presence of shock, extreme faecal contamination, extensive tissue damage, associated injuries, delay in operating after injury, and gross faecal loading.

Good results are now claimed in many centres from the use of primary closure in selected cases. It is agreed that patients with heavily contaminated wounds who present late with shock and numerous other injuries are best treated by colostomy, and that when contamination is minimal, there is a single injury, and presentation in early primary closure is feasible. The controversy rests with the cases that fall between these categories.

Specific injuries

Swallowed objects

Sharp ingested objects may travel with the faeces and lacerate the bowel or anal mucosa. Fish and chicken bones have been implicated, along with various more obscure objects in patients with psychiatric conditions. Patients may present with acute anal pain, and an acute anal fissure may be wrongly diagnosed. A careful anorectal examination, which may need to be performed under anaesthesia, will enable diagnosis and allow removal of the offending object.

Foreign bodies in the rectum

The introduction of foreign bodies through the anus is not as common as the prevalence of medical anecdotes suggests. Numerous objects have been described, including bottles, light bulbs, fruits, broom handles, vibrators, and other phallic objects. They are usually inserted deliberately, either by the patient or their partner, for erotic stimulation, but objects are also introduced during drunken play acting and assaults. Rectal lacerations are seen after fist fornication, when the fist is inserted into the rectum for sexual gratification. Rectal thermometers and enema nozzles are occasionally mislaid in the rectum.

Most foreign bodies can be removed through the anus under anaesthesia. This is facilitated by anal dilatation and applying pressure with a hand in the suprapubic region. After removal of the object the rectum is examined for underlying injury, although full thickness tears are unusual. Laparotomy and open removal of the foreign body is rarely necessary.

Obstetric injury

A perineal tear caused by parturition is a common anorectal injury, in which the anal sphincter mechanism is damaged. Immediate repair of the sphincter gives the best result. If this is not done, or if sepsis develops, the anal sphincter may be compromised, resulting in incontinence.

Iatrogenic injury

The rectum may be perforated by a sigmoidoscope or enema nozzle. This is largely preventable if care is taken and should

> **Contraindications to primary repair or resection and anastomosis**
>
> - Shock
> - Extreme faecal contamination
> - Extensive tissue damage
> - Associated injuries
> - Delay in operating after injury
> - Gross faecal loading

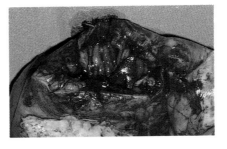

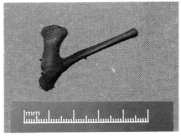

Fig 22.5 Perforation of the terminal ileum (upper) caused by chicken bone (lower).

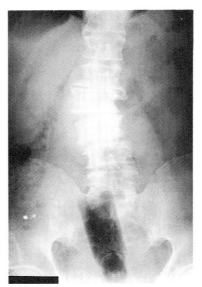

Fig 22.6 Radiograph showing roll on deodorant bottle in the rectum.

be a rare occurrence. Biopsy specimens of tumours can be taken safely, but mucosal biopsy specimens taken with the large rigid biopsy forceps should be taken only within 10 cm of the anus because of the risk of perforation.

Dilatation of rectal strictures and diathermy or laser treatment of rectal tumours may cause perforation. Urethral dilatation causing a false passage or open prostatectomy may damage the anterior wall of the rectum.

An iatrogenic injury is usually recognised at the time of occurrence. Immediate closure of a perforation and formation of a defunctioning colostomy is recommended. Minor injuries can be managed conservatively with active observation and antibiotics.

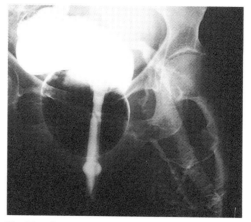

Fig 22.7 Barium enema radiograph showing contrast tracking into the buttock after rectal perforation.

Impalement

Impalement injuries are usually accidental. Falls on to railings or pitchforks may cause severe damage with little external evidence of injury if the object enters through the anus. The seat of a BMX bicycle and of a surgeon's operating room stool have been reported to have caused such rectal tramua.

Pneumatic injury

A compressed air nozzle applied to the rectum as a practical joke may cause colonic perforation. Patients present with signs of an intra-abdominal catastrophe and require resuscitation and urgent laparotomy.

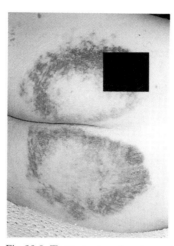

Fig 22.8 Torn, ruptured rectum with bruising of the buttocks caused by self abuse. (Identifying feature is masked.)

Pelvic fractures

The rectum may be punctured by bone fragments after major pelvic fracture, when there will usually be coincident bladder, prostate, and urethral injuries. Bone fragments and dislocation of the prostate are felt on rectal examination. A defunctioning colostomy or Hartmann type resection is indicated.

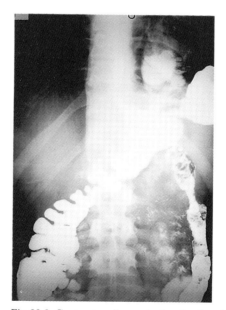

Fig 22.9 Contrast radiograph showing herniation of colon and stomach into the thorax caused by rupture of the diaphragm after blunt abdominal trauma.

The radiographs were provided by Dr Maeve McPhillips (Chinese University of Hong Kong), Mr P Plunkett (St James Hospital, Dublin), and Dr Brian Hourihane (St Vincent's Hospital, Dublin).

23   Sexually transmitted diseases and anal papillomas

B P Goorney

A variety of infections may be transmitted during anal intercourse, which is predominantly a practice of homosexual men, but also may affect some heterosexuals. It is important to consider the possibility of sexually transmitted disease in patients presenting with anorectal disorders and seek the advice of a genitourinary physician in appropriate cases.

Common anorectal sexually transmitted infections

- Gonococcus infection
- Chlamydia infection
- Herpes
- Primary syphilis

Gonorrhoea

Gonorrhoea is caused by *Neisseria gonorrhoea*, a Gram negative diplococcus. The organism is spread during anal intercourse and by autocontamination from the vagina in women. An incubation period of 5–7 days is followed by proctitis and infection of the anal crypts. Patients with symptomatic disease have pruritus ani, mucopurulent discharge, tenesmus, and bleeding. Disseminated infections may be associated with systemic manifestations including joint pains.

Most people with rectal gonorrhoea are, however, asymptomatic. About a quarter of homosexual men with gonorrhoea have anorectal involvement.

Proctoscopy shows proctitis, and mucopus can often be expressed from the anal crypts. The anal canal itself is usually spared. Swabs are taken for microscopic examination and culture to confirm the diagnosis.

Infected patients are treated with amoxycillin or, if they are allergic to penicillin, with either ciprofloxacin or spectinomycin. Treatment may start before obtaining positive cultures if there is a strong suspicion of gonorrhoea.

Patients should be screened at two weeks after treatment to confirm eradication of the infection. Sexual contacts should be traced, screened, and treated.

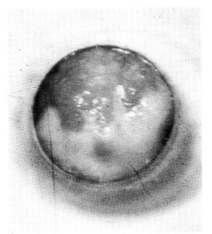

Fig 23.1 Gonococcal proctitis with considerable purulent rectal discharge.

Anal syphilis

An anal chancre is a common manifestation of primary syphilis. Three quarters of those infected are homosexual men. The chancre appears 2–6 weeks after exposure during anal intercourse. It may be confused with an anal fissure and when secondary bacterial infection supervenes can cause considerable pain at the anus.

Most patients with primary anal syphilis have painless inguinal lymphadenopathy, which is rare in patients with anal fissures. Early lesions are teeming with spirochaetes, which are readily shown by dark field microscopy.

The fluorescent treponemal antibody test (FTA) is the first serological test to become positive, 4–6 weeks after infection. The Venereal Disease Research Laboratory (VDRL) assay gives positive results in three quarters of patients with primary syphilis. The *Treponema pallidum* haemagglutination assay (TPHA) is also useful as a specific confirmatory test.

Secondary syphilis appears usually 6–8 weeks after the primary lesion. Patients develop moist, smooth, warty masses around the anus (condylomata lata) and have a discharge and pruritus. The warts are less keratinised, smoother, flatter, and moister than anal papillomas. These lesions are highly

Characteristics of anal syphilis

Primary syphilis
Anal chancre
Inguinal lymphadenopathy
Lesions infected with spirochaetes

Secondary syphilis
Condylomata lata
Lesions infected with spirochaetes

Tertiary syphilis
Rectal gumma
Tabes dorsalis
Severe perianal pain
Paralysis of sphincters

infectious because spirochaetes are abundant in the discharge. Condylomata lata may develop in any patient with secondary syphilis irrespective of the site of the primary lesion. All three serological tests for syphilis usually give positive results.

Tertiary syphilis is now rare. Rectal gumma may be confused with malignancy and patients with tabes dorsalis may have severe perianal pain and functional problems caused by paralysis of the sphincters.

Patients with syphilis are treated with intramuscular penicillin. Those allergic to penicillin are treated with tetracycline or erythromycin. Follow up serological tests are repeated periodically for at least a year after treatment to confirm eradication of the infection.

Chlamydia infection

Chlamydia trachomatis infection is a cause of proctitis among those who practice anoreceptive intercourse and may be subclinical. There are two strains or biovars: *Chlamydia trachomatis* and *Chlamydia lymphogranuloma venereum*. Symptoms include a mucoid or blood stained discharge, pain, tenesmus, and fever. Those with lymphogranuloma venereum may have inguinal lymphadenopathy.

The pathogen is intracellular and difficult to show even on culture of rectal biopsy specimens. The cell culture and direct immunofluorescence assay are the most sensitive tests for chlamydial infection.

Infected patients and those with a strong likelihood of chlamydial infection are treated with tetracycline or erythyromycin or a prolonged course of vibramycin. Rectal stricture is a rare complication of lymphogranuloma venereum as a result of L1-3 serovars; however, this rarely requires surgical treatment.

Herpes simplex virus

Herpes simplex virus infection is common among homosexual men and is an important complication of HIV infection. Chronic mucocutaneous herpes simplex virus infection in a patient infected with HIV is considered diagnostic for AIDS, particularly if it is of the ulcerative and persistent variety (more than a month's duration). Ninety per cent of anal infections are caused by herpes simplex virus type 2 and 10% by type 1. Symptoms develop 1–3 weeks after anal intercourse and include burning, mucoid or bloody discharge, and constitutional symptoms such as malaise and fever. Examination reveals vesicles, pustules, and shallow ulcers around the anus. Sigmoidoscopy shows proctitis and pronounced erythema. The lesions are usually extremely sore, precluding examination without an anaesthetic.

Infection can be confirmed by viral culture of vesicular fluid.

Patients are treated with oral or intravenous acyclovir depending on the severity of the illness. Treatment is continued until all the mucocutaneous surfaces have healed.

Human immunodeficiency virus

Many patients with HIV infection have anorectal problems, such as haemorrhoids, fissures, fistulas, and perianal abscesses, which may present as a first indication of AIDS.

Cytomegalovirus

Cytomegalovirus is a common secondary infection in patients with AIDS. The most important coloproctological manifestation is ileocolitis, which affects 10%. Patients present with severe diarrhoea, pain, and tenderness and constitutional disturbances. They may have perianal ulcers and typically

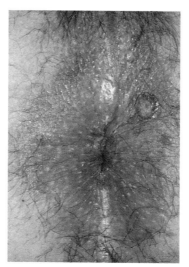

Fig 23.2 Primary syphilitic ulcer at the anal margin. These ulcers are often painful and tender.

Symptoms of acute proctitis

- Pruritis ani
- Anal discharge
- Anal pain
- Rectal bleeding
- Diarrhoea

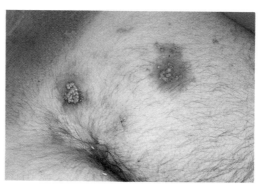

Fig 23.3 Anal herpes: the external vesicular lesions are characteristic of primary anorecal herpes simplex.

Proctocolitis associated with HIV and AIDS

Protozoa
  Cryptosporidia
  Isospora belli
  Entamoeba histolytica
  Microsporidia

Bacteria
  Mycobacterium avium-intracellulare
  Salmonella, Shigella spp.
  Campylobacter sp.

Viruses
  Cytomegalovirus
  Enteric viruses

---

have proctitis. Biopsy specimens of ulcers are taken to look for cytomegalic intranuclear inclusion bodies and for viral culture. Histological examination may show characteristic cytomegalovirus inclusion bodies. The condition is easily confused clinically with ulcerative colitis or Crohn's disease. Rarely patients may have bleeding or perforation of an ulcer, which carries a high risk of death.

Ganciclovir, an antiviral agent, is currently the best available treatment for cytomegalovirus infection. Foscarnet may also be used. Surgery is very rarely necessary for bleeding or perforation.

Cryptosporidiosis

Cryptosporidium may cause life threatening colitis in patients with AIDS. It causes severe enterocolitis with profuse secretory diarrhoea. Oocytes may be shown in the stool or rectal biopsy specimens. Patients require resuscitation, and antiparasitic treatment with paromomycin may be helpful.

Isosporiasis

Isosporiasis is another opportunistic infection, which causes enterocolitis with diarrhoea, vomiting, fever, and abdominal pain. The diagnosis is made by a modified fast acid stain of fresh stool. This infection responds well to co-trimoxazole, but maintenance therapy is usually required.

Microsporidiosis

An opportunistic protozoal infection is usually diagnosed using Giemsa staining. There is no specific treatment, but albendazole has been used.

Mycobacterium avium-intracellulare

Intestinal infection with *Mycobacterium avium-intracellulare* may present as diarrhoea with abdominal pain. The organisms are resistant to most conventional treatment and therapy usually includes clarithromycin and rifabutin. Some patients develop considerable mesenteric lymphadenopathy, which produces a characteristic doughy feeling on abdominal examination. It may be sufficient to cause bowel obstruction.

Other enteric infections

Other enteric infections, such as with *Entamoeba histolytica*, *Shigella* spp., *Salmonella* spp., and *Campylobacter* spp., can cause proctocolitis and may be acquired through the oral–anal route. *Giardia lamblia* may be difficult to diagnose and empirical therapy with metronidazole is effective.

Enteric viruses

This group of viruses, including adenovirus and rotavirus has been reported to cause a self limiting diarrhoea. Diagnosis is usually confirmed by electron microscopy of stool or a gut biopsy sample. There is no specific treatment.

Opportunistic tumours

Kaposi's sarcoma affecting the gastrointestinal tract may present with perianal, rectal, or colonic lesions. Most are asymptomatic, but occasionally they cause obstruction or bleeding. Surgical resection is rarely necessary.

Anorectal surgery

Asymptomatic patients with HIV infection tolerate colorectal surgery well. Morbidity is increased and wound healing often delayed in CDC stage III, persistent generalised lymphadenopathy, and CDC IV. Caution is advised before performing major anorectal surgery in these patients, although the final decision will depend on the patient's disease and condition.

Fig 23.4 The presence of acid fast bacilli in a stool specimen is helpful in the diagnosis of *Mycobacterium avium-intracellulare* infection.

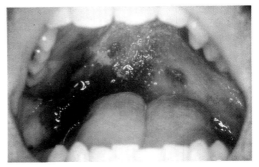

Fig 23.5 Kaposi's sarcoma of the palate. Many patients will have gastrointestinal involvement, which is often asymptomatic.

Investigation of proctocolitis

- Perform stool microscopy and culture
  —For protozoa and bacteria (that is, with acid fast staining for *Cryptosporidium* spp. and atypical mycobacteria)
- Take rectal specimens
  —For viruses and signs of other sexually transmitted diseases (for example, herpes simplex)
- Perform sigmoidoscopy and rectal biopsy
  —For cytomegalovirus and Kaposi's sarcoma

Anal papillomas

Anal papillomas are relatively common and are increasing in incidence. They are of viral origin, being caused by infection with human papilloma virus, notably types 6, 16, and 11. There is an increased incidence among homosexual men who practice anoreceptive intercourse, suggesting a venereal mode of transmission. Anal papillomas also arise, however, in the absence of anal sexual contact among heterosexual men and women.

The papillomas appear as white, pink, or grey lesions around the anus and perineum and inside the anal canal. There may be associated lesions on the penis and vulva. They vary greatly in number and extent from a few small scattered papillomas to bulky lesions without discernible intervening skin. The symptoms vary accordingly; they include itching, discomfort, discharge, and bleeding. Many people with anal papillomas do not have any symptoms.

They can be self limiting and resolve spontaneously after several years, perhaps owing to an effective host immune response.

The lesions are usually obvious on inspection of the perineum. Proctoscopy should be performed systematically to identify lesions within the anal canal and rectum which may require treatment. Many patients will have other anogenital sexually transmitted diseases and so all patients should be fully screened for other sexually transmitted diseases.

Treatment

Several different methods of treatment have been described and should be adapted to the individual patient.

Repeated application of chemical agents such as podophyllin is suitable for small numbers of polyps outside the anal canal if they are of viral origin. Warts persisting after a month are unlikely to respond to further applications.

Persistent and more extensive warts are treated by surgical excision or ablation by diathermy. Infiltration of the affected area with a weak solution of adrenaline helps show the individual lesions, which can be picked off with a fine scalpel, preserving the intervening skin. Coagulation by using diathermy or laser is also effective but causes greater discomfort afterwards.

Recurrence is common so it is important to treat coexistent genital lesions and sexual partners. Advice about barrier contraception should be given where appropriate.

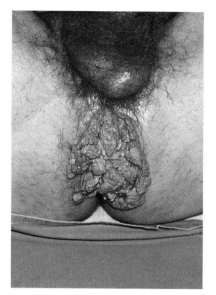

Fig 23.6 Anal warts extending into the anal canal.

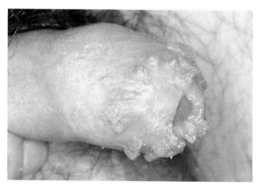

Fig 23.7 Genital warts: secondary spread to the anal region is not uncommon.

24 Tropical colonic diseases

B K Mandal, P F Schofield

In this age of increasing foreign travel it is quite possible for a patient presenting with diarrhoea to be suffering from a tropically acquired infection. Unless an accurate travel history is taken the diagnosis may be delayed with a resultant increase in morbidity caused by inappropriate treatment.

Either the small or the large bowel may be affected (and occasionally both). A good history of the nature of the diarrhoea often allows differentiation between these two sites. Small bowel diarrhoea is usually of large volume, watery, and devoid of blood and mucus whereas, when the large bowel is affected the stools are of small volume, are frequent, may be associated with tenesmus, and are often bloody.

In large bowel diarrhoea, if visible blood is not present, a faecal smear will generally disclose pus cells and red blood cells. This is because, whereas most small bowel diarrhoea is caused by enterotoxin producing organisms, the organisms that affect the large bowel are invasive and lead to colorectal inflammation. Some organisms affect both the large and the small bowel.

Amoebic dysentery

Amoebic dysentery is a relatively rare import. The clinical picture is typically that of a gradually worsening diarrhoea, which if untreated persists for a few weeks then subsides but may recur at irregular intervals. The stools are liquid, faecal, and bloody. The diagnosis may be missed unless fresh warm stools are examined promptly to show the characteristically motile amoebic trophozoites with ingested red blood cells. The amoebas stop moving on cooling and assume a round shape in stale stool specimens and thus become difficult to identify. In less severe cases the diagnosis is best achieved by prompt microscopy of the curettage material obtained during endoscopy.

Although the presence of typical amoebic ulcers with undermined edges and intervening normal mucosa will facilitate clinical diagnosis, the appearance at sigmoidoscopy is often indistinguishable from other causes of colitis—infective or non-infective. A high index of suspicion is necessary as injudicious use of corticosteroids may have disastrous consequences.

Treatment

Metronidazole 800 mg three times a day for five days will usually effect a prompt clinical cure, but a luminal amoebicide such as diloxanide furoate 0·5 g three times a day for five days is needed to eradicate the infection.

Bacillary dysentry

Bacillary dysentery is caused by shigella organisms. Of the four recognised species of *Shigella* (*Sh. sonnei*, *Sh. flexneri*, *Sh. dysenteriae*, *Sh. boydii*), *Sh. sonnei* is most common in Britain, but tropically acquired infections are usually caused by *Sh. flexneri* and occasionally. *Sh. dysenteriae* type 1 (Shiga's bacillus). The resultant illness is usually more severe than Sonne dysentery, with numerous bloody stools and pronounced tenesmus. Dysentery caused by *Sh. dysenteriae* may be complicated by the development of necrotising enterocolitis with toxic megacolon or perforation.

Examples of diarrhoea causing organisms acquired in tropical countries

Small bowel
Vibrio cholerae
Enterotoxigenic *Escherichia coli*
Vibrio parahaemolyticus
Giardia species
Cryptosporidium species

Large bowel
Entamoeba histolytica
Balantidium coli
Enteroinvasive *E. coli*
Clostridium difficile
Schistosoma species

Small bowel and large bowel
Shigella species
Salmonella species
Campylobacter species
Plesiomonas shigelloides
Aeromonas hydrophila
Yersinia enterocolita

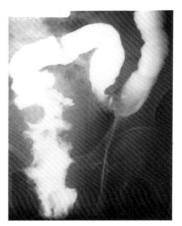

Fig 24.1 Barium enema radiograph in a patient with bloody mucoid diarrhoea showing amoebic ulceration. Two stool examinations yielded negative results but fresh endoscopic biopsy specimens proved positive for motile amoebas.

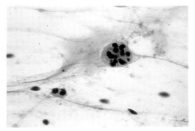

Fig 24.2 Photomicrograph of *Entamoeba histolytica* showing engulfed red blood cells (trichrome stain; magnification ×480).

90

Antibiotics are indicated for severe shigella dysentery. The organisms are often resistant to commonly used antibiotics such as ampicillin and co-trimoxazole. One of the 4-quinolones, ciprofloxacin, is the drug of choice in adults, but in children 4-quinolones are not generally used because of their propensity to cause damage to cartilage in growing animals (this has not been reported in humans). Nalidixic acid or other antibiotics may be used instead but guidance about sensitivity of the bacteria is important. Rarely, patients require an operation for perforative disease.

Salmonella and campylobacter enterocolitis

Salmonella and campylobacter organisms are common causes of bacterial diarrhoea worldwide and may affect a traveller to a tropical country. The illness begins abruptly with fever, headache, vomiting, and colicky abdominal pain and the passage of large volume, watery, often bloodstained stools, but at times the motions are frankly bloody owing to prominent colonic involvement. Ileocaecal involvement may mimic appendicitis. The presence of toxic dilatation or segmental colitis may confuse the diagnosis by suggesting underlying non-specific inflammatory bowel disease.

Sigmoidoscopy has limited discriminatory value in differentiating infective colitis from inflammatory bowel disease. Early rectal biopsy may not be helpful in distinguishing between infective colitis and the initial presentation of inflammatory bowel disease because the histological features associated with ulcerative colitis are often clearly seen only after some weeks. Repeat biopsy 6–10 weeks after the onset of symptoms will, however, usually clarify the diagnostic dilemma because by this time either the appearances will have resolved or features of chronicity will have become apparent.

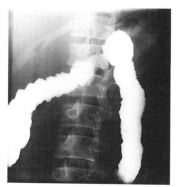

Fig 24.3 Barium enema radiograph in a returning traveller with bloody diarrhoea showing colitis. Sigmoidoscopy showed florid colitis. Ulcerative colitis was initially suspected because of two negative stool cultures but this third stool specimen proved positive for *Sh. flexneri*.

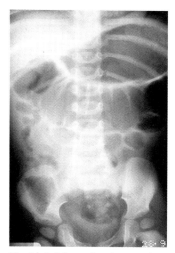

Fig 24.4 Megacolon in a patient with salmonella colitis.

Histological features in acute and chronic colitis

	Acute colitis	Chronic ulcerative colitis
Cellular infiltrate		
Polymorphs	+ +	±
Mononuclear	±	+ +
Distortion of crypts	−	+ +
Mucus depletion	±	+ +

The diagnosis of intestinal schistosomiasis is based on showing the presence of eggs in faeces or in rectal biopsy specimens

Treatment

Antibiotics are not usually indicated for salmonella or campylobacter infections. The illnesses are short lived and usually settling by the time of bacteriological diagnosis. Bacteraemia often complicates salmonella infections in elderly people and young children, however, and these patients should receive antibiotics. Patients with severe enterocolitis should also be treated. For salmonellosis ciprofloxacin is the drug of choice in adults, but in children a third generation cephalosporin such as cefotaxime may be used. (Ciprofloxacin is useful in eradicating the organisms in carriers of salmonellae.)

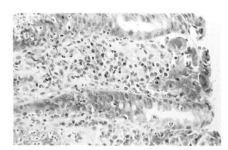

Fig 24.5 Histological slide of a rectal biopsy specimen showing proctitis in a patient with campylobacter infection (haematoxylin and eosin stain; magnification ×75).

In cases of campylobacteriosis erythromycin is the drug of choice, although ciprofloxacin is equally effective.

Schistosomiasis

There are three common schistosoma organisms. *Schistosoma haematobium* affects the bladder, but the large bowel venules are the preferred site for laying eggs by the adult females of both *Sch. mansoni*, prevalent in Africa, the Caribbean, and South America, and *Sch. japonicum*, prevalent in large parts of south east Asia. The trapped eggs in the tissues lead to granulomatous reaction. Most patients have few or no symptoms, though some may have mild diarrhoea with blood in the early stages.

In severe infection granulomas in the large bowel mucosa may develop into visible polyps, which may ulcerate and later produce dysentery like symptoms. In longstanding and recurrent infections the liver becomes enlarged from the large number of eggs reaching it through the portal circulation. This ultimately leads to hepatic fibrosis, portal hypertension, and splenomegaly.

Treatment

Praziquantel is effective in all forms of schistosomiasis and is the treatment of choice. It is given as a single dose of 40 mg/kg.

Rare infective colitides

Yersinia enterocolitica is a fairly common cause of acute diarrhoea in many parts of the world, including the tropics, but is quite uncommon in Britain. Enteritis or ileitis are the usual manifestations, but colonic inflammation may be present. The diagnosis is made by isolating the organism from the faeces or by showing there are antibodies to it in the serum.

Certain strains of *Escherichia coli* are invasive (enteroinvasive *E. coli*) and may produce a dysentery like picture. Their prevalence in the tropics is unclear.

Enterohaemorrhagic strains of *Escherichia coli*, in particular *E. coli* 0157 have emerged as an important cause of bloody diarrhoea in many Western countries. Consumption of infected cattle and sheep products is usually responsible. Enteroinvasive strains of *E. coli* are another cause of dysentery like diarrhoea. Prevalence of these strains of *E. coli* in the tropics is unknown.

Plesiomonas shigelloides and *Aeromonas hydrophila* have recently joined the growing list of organisms known to be capable of producing colitis and can be contracted in the tropics as well as in temperate climates.

Cryptosporidium species has also recently emerged as a common cause of diarrhoea worldwide. They are protozoa which primarily affect the small intestine, causing watery diarrhoea, but may also be seen in rectal biopsy specimens.

Balantidium coli is a common parasite of animals which may rarely produce ulcerative colonic disease in humans.

In sexually active homosexual men, rectal discharge may result from proctitis caused by gonococcal, chlamydial, or herpes simplex (normally associated with perianal vesicles) infections acquired abroad. Gonococci in far eastern countries are often multi-drug resistant, even including ciprofloxacin.

Chronic diseases

Tuberculosis

Tuberculosis must be suspected in Asians with abdominal pain and chronic diarrhoea. It most commonly affects the ileocaecum and requires differentiation from Crohn's disease. The rectum may be affected and the disease may present as an ischiorectal abscess or ulcerative proctocolitis.

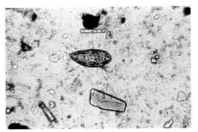

Fig 24.6 *Schistosoma mansoni* eggs in faeces. Note the typical lateral spine (magnification ×480).

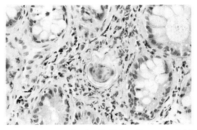

Fig 24.7 Histological slide of a rectal biopsy specimen in a patient with *Schistosoma mansoni* infection showing a trapped egg (haematoxylin and eosin stain; magnification ×75).

Causes of infective colitis

Salmonella species
Shigella species
Campylobacter species
Entamoeba histolytica
Balantidium coli
Enterohaemorrhagic *Escherichia coli*
Enteroinvasive *Escherichia coli*
Clostridium difficile
Plesiomonas shigelloides
Aeromonas hydrophila
Yersinia enterocolitica
Mycobacterium tuberculosis
Gonococci
Chlamydia species
Cytomegalovirus
Herpes simplex virus

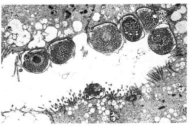

Fig 24.8 Electron micrograph of a rectal biopsy specimen in a patient with crytposporidial diarrhoea. The organisms are on the cell surface (magnification ×5500).

Chagas' disease

Chagas' disease is endemic in Brazil and in other areas of South America. The parasites destroy the ganglion cells of the gut, resulting in enteromegaly, in particular megaoesophagus and megacolon. Chronic progressive dysphagia and constipation are the usual manifestations and are often present for several years before the typical dilatation occurs.

The heart is commonly affected, leading to cardiomegaly and arrhythmia, which may result in sudden death.

Lymphogranuloma venereum

Lymphogranuloma venereum is a sexually transmitted disease, prevalent in the tropics and subtropics, caused by chlamydia group A organisms. Genital ulcers and associated painful inguinal glands, which may suppurate, are the usual presenting features, but proctitis may develop later and produce fibrotic rectal strictures. Formation of a perirectal abscess or a fistula may complicate the picture.

The diagnosis is usually made by serological testing or isolation of the organism, or both. Tetracycline controls the infection but surgery may be necessary in patients with chronic disease with suppurative or fibrotic complications.

HIV related

Chronic diarrhoea is a frequent problem in HIV infected patients. Globally the common causes are *Cryptosporidium* spp., *Microsporidium* spp., *Mycobacterium avium-intracellular* complex, cytomegalovirus (CMV), and herpes simplex virus (HSV), whereas *Isospora belli*, *Cyclospora* and *Mycobacterium tuberculosis* are additional causes in the tropics. CMV and HSV affect the colorectum, presenting as inflammatory colitis with bloody diarrhoea (CMV) or ulcerative anoproctitis with perianal vesicles (HSV). Other infections usually affect the small gut.

Differential diagnosis

Relapse of diarrhoea in a returned traveller may result from colitis caused by *Clostridium difficile* after taking antibiotics while abroad either as prophylaxis or for treating traveller's diarrhoea.

It should not be forgotten that diarrhoea in patients returning from the tropics may have non-infective causes. Each year we see examples of carcinoma of the colon, ulcerative colitis, Crohn's disease, and diverticulitis presenting as diarrhoea after foreign travel. Furthermore, the presence of an infective organism may be a concurrent event. In patients with persisting bloody diarrhoea underlying inflammatory bowel disease should be considered.

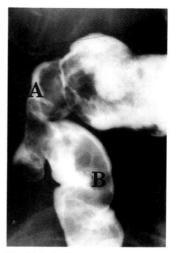

Fig 24.9 Barium enema radiograph in a patient with hypertrophic ileocaecal tuberculosis. Note the shortening of the ascending colon (A) and the dilated ileum (B).

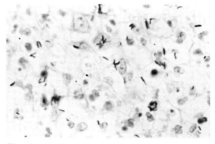

Fig 24.10 Black and white photomicrograph of tuberculosis caecum. Organisms are shown as black rods (Zeihl–Neelsen stain)—they would be red in a colour reproduction.

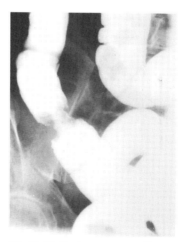

Fig 24.11 Barium enema radiograph showing carcinoma of the colon. This patient presented with diarrhoea after foreign travel and hence was suspected of having a tropical infection.

We thank Dr G C Cook for providing the photomicrograph of *Ent. histolytica* and the picture of *Sch. mansoni* eggs.

25 Paediatric problems

C M Doig

Some anorectal problems, such as constipation and anal fissure are common in both children and adults. Congenital problems such as anorectal agenesis and Hirschsprung's disease present in early infancy. Despite treatment in childhood the sequelae may require continuing management in adult life.

Constipation

Constipation is one of the most common causes of abdominal pain in childhood. A full rectum may compress the bladder, causing urinary problems. Constipation may be considered as either the passage of hard stools or an irregular bowel habit. Less easily recognisable is the passage of only small motions each day with the child retaining faeces. A palpable colon may be found on examination, but if the motion is soft radiography of the abdomen may be necessary to make the diagnosis.

If untreated three problems may arise: abdominal pain, anal fissure, and soiling because of overflow incontinence. The cause of constipation may be an inadequate diet, poor toilet facilities at home or more commonly at school, or previous illness or fever. Treatment involves dietary advice and toilet retraining. It may be necessary to empty the bowel by means of rectal washouts or enemas, or both, before giving laxatives, the dosage of which varies with each child. The general principles of treatment with laxatives include giving an adequate dosage for a long enough period of time, with gradual tailing off. Rarely a child may need admission to hospital for retraining.

Anal fissure—This is indicated by a history of pain on defecation with crying and "holding back" when on the toilet. Streaks of blood may be seen on toilet paper or the stool. A skin tag (sentinal pile) may indicate a fissure. Rectal examination should not be attempted if the diagnosis is obvious. Treatment entails oral laxatives for the constipation and applying local anaesthetic cream to the area. Suppositories should not be used. Occasionally anal stretch under general anaesthetic may be necessary to relieve sphincter spasm.

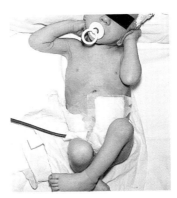
Fig 25.1 Infant with temporary caecostomy.

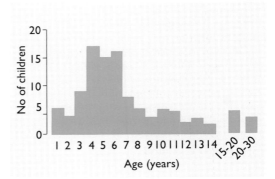
Fig 25.2 Age of children presenting with "idiopathic" constipation.

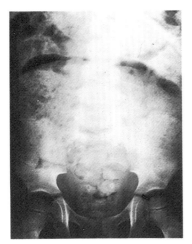
Fig 25.3 Abdominal radiograph showing severe constipation.

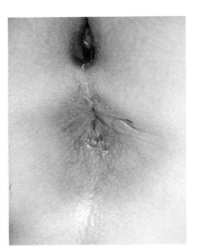
Fig 25.4 The anal tag is not the cause of the pain—it indicates the anal fissure, which is.

94

Rectal prolapse—This occurs in children under the age of 3 years. Cystic fibrosis must be excluded by a sweat test and massive intussusception can be excluded by rectal examination. By treating the constipation and reassuring the parents the prolapse will eventually cure itself. Surgery to fix the prolapse is rarely necessary.

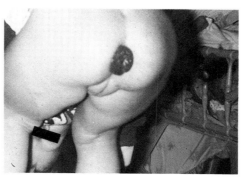

Fig 25.5 Rectal prolapse in an infant.

Hirschsprung's disease

Any child who has had constipation since birth, irrespective of age, may have Hirschsprung's disease. The disease presents either in a neonate as large bowel obstruction or later as chronic constipation. The diagnosis should be considered and excluded in any child who does not pass meconium for 48 hours or who passes a meconium plug only after rectal examination or insertion of a thermometer. The diagnosis should be considered in all constipated children, especially if constipation starts from birth or with delay in the passage of meconium. Soiling and faeces in the rectum may indicate that the disease is of short length. There is a lack of ganglion cells in Auerbach's plexus for varying lengths of bowel proximal from the anus. Total lack of ganglion cells throughout the colon or even the small bowel can occur. In children with very short or short affected segments the disease may not be diagnosed until they are teenagers. Anorectal manometry may be helpful in making the diagnosis in these children.

Diagnosis

Although it is a congenital disease, two thirds of children may be diagnosed after the age of 6 months. The diagnosis depends on radiological and histological findings. A barium enema examination is performed on the unprepared bowel. A plain abdominal radiograph 24 hours later showing retention of barium is highly suggestive. Biopsy specimens are taken from the rectum either at laparotomy or through the anus to give absolute proof—that is, the absence of ganglion cells. Histological examination of a punch biopsy specimen of mucosa and submucosa will exclude the disease if ganglion cells are present. Acetylcholinesterase activity may also be measured in these small specimens.

Treatment

The initial treatment to deflate the bowel is colostomy, which can either be in the right transverse colon if the stoma is created blind or at the junction of ganglionic and aganglionic bowel if laparotomy has been necessary to confirm the diagnosis. Although some surgeons favour deflation by rectal washouts and early neonatal definitive surgery, the usual practice is for colostomy in neonates followed by excision of aganglionic bowel and renastomosis. There are a variety of operations ("pull throughs") to reanastomose the ganglionic bowel to the normally innervated anus. The colostomy is left in place if it is in the right transverse colon and closed when the anastomosis is satisfactory or redone at surgery to divert faeces until the anastomosis is healed.

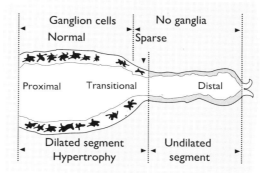

Fig 25.6 Histopathology of Hirschsprung's disease—the proximal colon is dilated and hypertrophied with ganglion cells becoming sparse at the transitional area and absent at the undilated (but not narrow) distal colon. The anus never has ganglion cells.

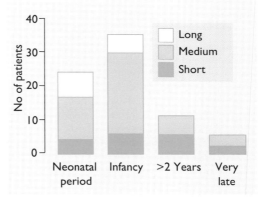

Fig 25.7 Age at presentation in relation to length of segment. (Numbers were obtained in the 1970s in London.)

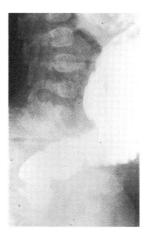

Fig 25.8 Barium enema radiograph showing cone at the transitional area with normal peristaltic dilated bowel to the aganglionic non-peristaltic normal sized bowel distally.

Complications

The major complication and most common cause of death in children with Hirschsprung's disease is enterocolitis which, although more common in infancy, may occur in older children with untreated Hirschsprung's disease. It presents as a fulminating infection (often clostridial in origin) with toxaemia, abdominal distension, and diarrhoea. Despite treatment with antibiotics, intravenous fluids, or even steroids and emergency colostomy, a third of these children die. Those who survive a stormy illness will have permanent mucosal damage of both ganglionic and aganglionic bowel and an increased risk of complications such as stricture and leakage after surgery. After treatment of Hirschsprung's disease many children continue to have the problem of soiling or constipation, but this eventually clears up and over 90% of these children have normal bowel habits.

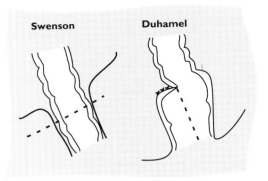

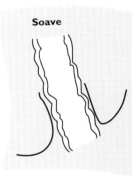

Fig 25.9 (a) Swenson operation—end to end anastomosis intussuscepting aganglionic and ganglionic bowel through anus and resection and anastomosis along dotted line. (b) Duhamel operation—anterior aganglionic and posterior ganglionic bowel. The dotted line indicates the stable closure and knife division between the two portions of bowel. (c) Soave operation—mucosa is removed, a muscular cuff of the aganglionic bowel is left and ganglionic bowel is pulled through to hang from the anus.

Rectal bleeding

Polyps

Painless bleeding suggests a solitary rectal polyp. These are almost always not adenomatous. The bleeding, separate from the stool and of moderate quantity, necessitates sigmoidoscopy and snaring of the polyp. Such polyps should be sent for histological examination to check that they are not premalignant. Multiple polyps elsewhere in the colon may require either flexible sigmoidoscopy or colonoscopy to make the diagnosis, for biopsy, and for treatment. Contrast barium enema examination can help to pinpoint the area. If the polyps are adenomatous follow up with repeated endoscopy is necessary. Polyposis coli can occur in children under 15 years, so follow up and treatment, even colectomy, may be necessary early.

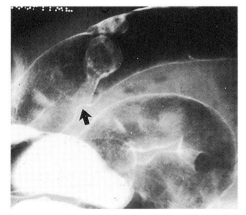

Fig 25.10 Contrast barium enema radiograph showing stalked polyp (arrowed) and more sessile polyp opposite.

Bright red bleeding through the anus usually indicates one of the following

- Anal fissure
- Rectal polyp
- Dysentery
- Inflammatory bowel disease

Intussusception

Intussusception occurs most commonly in infants 7–12 months old. In older children there is usually an associated polyp, diverticulum, or tumour. Although classically the diagnosis is made on the basis of colicky abdominal pain, a sausage shaped mass, and dark red blood through the rectum, 10% present with diarrhoea and vomiting suggestive of gastroenteritis. Bleeding through the rectum indicates that the bowel is compromised; it occurs in about half of the patients.

If the child is not in shock, which is often the case, barium or air enema examination may not only confirm the diagnosis but also treat the intussusception as the hydrostatic pressure can reduce the bowel. More often surgery has to be performed after resuscitation. If resection of the bowel is necessary the ileocaecal value and terminal ileum may be lost.

Meckel's diverticulum may present with bleeding because of an intussusception or because of the presence of gastric mucosa.

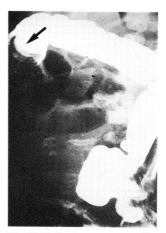

Fig 25.11 Barium enema radiograph showing intussusception in right transverse colon.

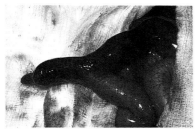

Fig 25.12 Meckel's diverticulum which has been involved in an intussusception.

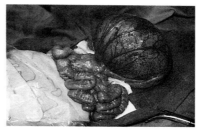

Fig 25.13 Duplication cyst of small bowel with flattened bowel.

Duplication cyst

Any part of the gastrointestinal tract may be duplicated; the colon is the part least commonly duplicated. The diagnosis is made by using ultrasonography and radiography to show displacement of the bowel. Spinal abnormalities—for example, hemivertebrae—can be associated, though not necessarily at the level of the abnormality. When a dupliction cyst occurs in a short portion of bowel it is usually possible to excise both the cyst and the segment of bowel affected, with reanastomosis of the colon.

Number of children in Britain with inflammatory bowel disease[1]	
• Crohn's disease	447
• Ulcerative colitis	305
• Other inflammatory bowel disease	34

Inflammatory bowel disease

Inflammatory bowel disease does occur in childhood. The number of children under the age of 12 years with Crohn's disease is increasing.

The presentation, diagnosis, and treatment of ulcerative colitis and Crohn's disease in children are similar to those in adults. Children may present with extragastrointestinal problems, such as arthritis, skin rashes, and uveitis, many months or years before abdominal pain, weight loss, and mouth ulcers make the diagnosis of Crohn's disease obvious. In addition to endoscopy and biopsy diagnosis has been improved by the use of small bowel enemas and sucralfate scans to pin point active areas.

Surgery for Crohn's disease in children, when performed early because of stunting of growth and failure of sexual development, has tended to give fewer immediate postoperative problems than in adults and may lead to a growth spurt, though the risk of recurrence is high.

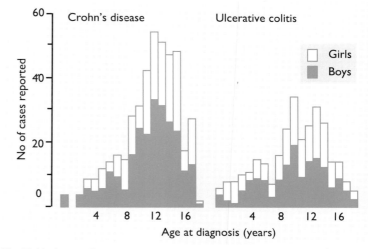

Fig 25.14 Age at diagnosis of Crohn's disease and ulcerative colitis.[1].

Anorectal anomalies

Anorectal anomalies are congenital abnormalities of either the anus or rectum, or both. The anus can be absent, abnormal, or ectopic. There are many different types of anomaly, which may or may not involve fistulous connections to skin, vagina, or urethra. The main distinction, however, is whether the bowel ends above or below the levator ani muscle. Isolated colonic atresia may also occur.

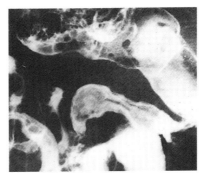

Fig 25.15 Small bowel barium enema radiograph in a child with Crohn's disease showing narrowed ileum just proximal to ileocaecal valve.

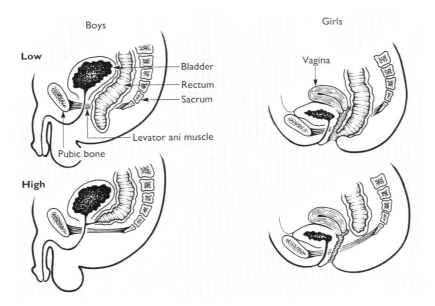

Fig 25.16 Common anorectal anomalies (a) in boys and (b) in girls, showing relationship in high and low anorectal abnormalities between bowel, levator ani muscle, skin, urethra, and vagina.

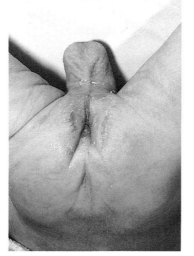

Fig 25.17 Male infant perineum with pin hole anus showing excoriation caused by passage of "toothpaste stools" as a result of delayed diagnosis.

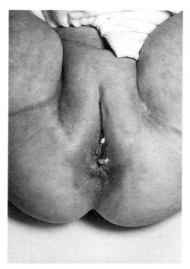

Fig 25.18 Female perineum showing anterior placed anus just inside the forchette.

The low type of anomaly includes those in which the bowel passes through a normal levator ani muscle to end blindly a few centimetres from the anus (imperforate anus) or enters the perineum in an abnormal position. The diagnosis is made by careful inspection of the perineum for a fistulous connection to skin on the penile shaft or median raphe of the scrotum in a boy or just within the vestibule in a girl. Treatment usually involves the deroofing of such a fistula by cutting back to a normal anus. Long term continence is ensured if the sphincter muscles are normal. Occasionally an anoplasty to place an ectopic anus in a normal position may be necessary. Early inspection of the perineum in babies to pick up an ectopic or stenotic anal opening improves long term outlook.

It is important that the high type of anorectal anomaly is not misdiagnosed as a low imperforate anus. In these children the bowel ends above the levator ani, which is often poorly developed. The distinction can be made by inspection and lateral inverted radiography performed 24 hours after birth to find out where the intestinal gas ends. Should gas appear not to reach the pubococcygeal line, a high type of anomaly is probable and perineal exploration should not be done.

Treatment may entail performing a colostomy with subsequent "pull through" of the colon through the pelvic muscles and involving the sphincter muscles present to the perineum. The earlier such reconstruction surgery is carried out the more likely the child will develop normal continence. Various operations have been developed using abdominal, sacral, and perineal approaches to reconstitute the anatomy. The most recent, a posterior approach dividing the muscles and tapering the colon before bringing it on to the perineum, has had promising early results.

As a result of poor or absent musculature children with high anomalies may be slow to gain continence, but by strenuous training to use such muscles as are present, tightening the muscles later by levatorplasty, giving advice about diet, and keeping the "neorectum" empty, improvement may occur. More than a half of children with any type of anorectal anomaly will have at least one other abnormality. In view of the high incidence of renal problems all of these children should have their urinary tract examined at an early age.

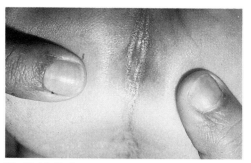

Fig 25.19 Perineum with no anus or fistula—probable high type anomaly.

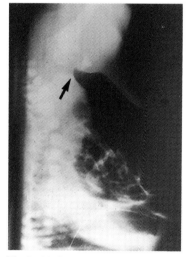

Fig 25.20 Inverted lateral radiograph showing intestinal gas just at level of coccyx–pubis line (high type anomaly).

The photographs were prepared by the medical illustration department, North Manchester General Hospital.

[1]Ferguson A, Rifkind E, Doig CM. Prevalence of chronic inflammatory bowel disease in British children. In: *Frontiers of gastrointestinal research*, vol 11. Basel: Karger, 1986:68–72.

Anomalies associated with colorectal problems in children

- Congenital heart disease — 12–20%
- Skeletal problems — 15–20%
- Tetralogy of Fallot and atresia 5–10%
- Other intestinal problems — 5%
- Urological problems — 30–50%

26   Drugs in the management of colorectal diseases

G L Carlson, J L Shaffer

Drugs used for diarrhoea

- Opiate and opiate related drugs
- Kaolin and chalk
- Bulking agents
- Bile salt binding agents
- Glucose and electrolyte mixtures.

Opiate related drugs

The chief opiate related drugs are codeine phosphate, loperamide, and diphenoxylate. These act on colonic opiate receptors to reduce colonic motility, although an effect on intestinal electrolyte absorption and secretion may also be relevant.

All of these preparations are highly effective in the management of acute diarrhoea. Loperamide (in small doses) is available without prescription but should be used as an adjunct to glucose and electrolyte mixtures.

Problems may arise with long term use of opiates: tolerance can occur with all three and dependence has been reported for diphenoxylate and codeine.

Diphenoxylate is available only in combination with atropine (co-phenotrope), which is added to reduce the risk of misuse. Unfortunately it also increases the incidence of adverse effects.

None of the preparations is recommended for use in children under four years of age.

Kaolin and chalk

Kaolin and chalk work by adsorbing water, which increases the viscosity of the stool. They are unpalatable, making them of little value in long term conditions. Combinations of kaolin and a small dose of morphine are available without prescription and are relatively inexpensive and safe. Clinical trials have failed to show any evidence of efficacy but they are popular in the management of acute diarrhoea.

Bulking agents

Bulking agents are conventionally thought of as laxatives, but they may be of value in long term diarrhoea. When taken with minimal water they thicken the stool, making diarrhoea more acceptable to some patients. They are useful in the early days after creation of a colostomy as they thicken the stoma effluent, making stoma training easier and increasing the patient's confidence.

Bile salt binding agents

Cholestyramine and aluminium hydroxide bind bile salts. The presence of bile salts within the colon may play a major part in the development of diarrhoea because of their osmotic and irritant effects. Causes include terminal ileal disease or resection. Early consideration should be given to this mechanism of diarrhoea as treatment with bile salt binding agents may be highly effective. The timing of cholestyramine administration is important. It must be taken with food and not one hour before or after food as is commonly advised. If other drugs are taken concurrently they may also bind to cholestyramine and thus they should be given at least one hour before or four hours after cholestyramine. The disadvantage of this form of treatment is that by binding bile salts fat malabsorption may be increased.

Glucose and electrolyte mixtures

The intestinal absorption of salt and water is considerably enhanced by the addition of glucose, and glucose and electrolyte mixtures act rapidly to reduce the loss of fluid which may complicate infective diarrhoea leading to potentially lethal dehydration, especially in the very young. They play an important part in the maintenance of fluid balance in infective diarrhoea in the United Kingdom and the newer, flavoured mixtures have the added attraction of being palatable, inexpensive, and free from adverse effects.

Several oral rehydration solutions are now available. They have similar electrolyte composition and choice should be led by patient preference. The solutions used in the United Kingdom are lower in sodium and higher in glucose than the WHO formulation. They are therefore of benefit only for mild to moderate diarrhoea, when the body's homoeostatic mechanisms are still working, but may be suboptimal for correcting severe fluid losses and electrolyte imbalance. It is important to appreciate that oral rehydration solution corrects fluid imbalance but does not reduce diarrhoea.

Aperients, suppositories, enemas, and bowel preparation

The chief laxative preparations available are traditionally divided into four categories

- Bulking agents
- Stimulant laxatives
- Faecal softeners
- Osmotic laxatives.

Bulking agents

Ispaghula husk, sterculia, bran, and methylcellulose all act on the colon by increasing the amount of indigestible residue in the stool. The hydrophilic nature of these compounds both softens the stool and increases volume. Flatulence and colicky pain may make them less acceptable to patients than other laxative preparations. The agents are formulated as powders (to be mixed as flavoured drinks), granules (to be ingested directly or added to food), and tablets. All of these preparations should be taken with water, but not immediately before going to bed as cases of intestinal obstruction have been reported under these circumstances.

Stimulant laxatives

Senna, bisacodyl, danthron, and docusate act by both increasing colonic motility and altering colonic fluid and electrolyte transport. These preparations are of value in the short term management of constipation associated with, for example, opiates in terminal care. They should be used as second line treatment after bulking agents. The increase in colonic motility may lead to colicky abdominal pain, so the preparations should be introduced gradually.

The use of danthron, available as co-danthramer and co-danthrusate, has been restricted because studies on rodents have indicated a potential risk of carcinogenicity. Use is now limited to the management of constipation in elderly patients, the prophylaxis and treatment of analgesic induced constipation in terminally ill patients, and for constipation complicating cardiac failure and myocardial infarction, where straining during defecation should be avoided. Controlled intermittent use of stimulants is to be preferred as continuous use results in tolerance and the risk of cathartic colon. Non-standardised preparations—cascara, frangula, rhubarb, and senna—should be avoided as the dose of the active ingredient is unpredictable.

Faecal softeners

In addition to docusate (which is also a stimulant) arachis oil and liquid paraffin have been extensively used to "soften" the faeces and relieve constipation. Oily preparations are almost obselete, with the exception of arachis oil enemas (which may be of value in elderly patients with intractable constipation).

Oral liquid paraffin preparations should be avoided as they cause anal irritation and reduced absorption of fat soluble vitamins. Systemic absorption also occurs, which may lead to a generalised granulomatous reaction and, rarely, lipid inhalation with resulting pulmonary injury (olegranuloma).

Osmotic laxatives

Osmotic laxatives reduce colonic absorption of fluid by an osmotic effect within the lumen of the bowel. Lactulose is one of the most popular laxatives but is expensive and is no more effective than the much less expensive magnesium salts. The main indication for lactulose is in hepatic encephalopathy.

Magnesium salts are highly effective but have become less popular in recent years. Magnesium absorption may result in toxicity, which can cause problems in patients with chronic renal failure.

Evacuant suppositories

Suppositories are useful alternative to oral preparations in chronic constipation, though acceptability to patients may be a problem. Glycerine preparations soften the stool and have a mild stimulant effect. Phosphate and citrate preparations act by an osmotic mechanism.

Bowel preparation

The aim of bowl preparation is to cleanse the bowel of residue. This is performed before colonoscopy, barium enema, and colorectal surgery, and occasionally as a last line of treatment for patients with intractable slow transit constipation. Phospahate enemas can cleanse the left colon. Both mannitol solution and Klean Prep—an isosmotic solution of polyethylene glycol—may be taken orally to produce a more thorough colonic cleansing.

Sodium picosulphate with magnesium citrate (Picolax) has both osmotic and stimulant properties and is inexpensive. Although whole gut irrigation with saline and potassium achieves excellent results, unacceptability to patients reduces its use.

These powerful agents may provoke significant fluid shifts and lead to substantial morbidity. They should be used with extreme caution in elderly patients and serum electrolyte concentrations should be monitored carefully.

Antispasmodic agents

A large number of drugs are available for treating "colonic spasm", which is believed to be a feature of the irritable bowel syndrome.

Antimuscarinic preparations (propantheline bromide, hyoscine butylbromide) reduce motility by antagonising the muscarinic cholinergic receptors on colonic smooth muscle. These preparations unfortunately have other anticholinergic actions and may lead to urinary retention, blurred vision and photophobia, acute glaucoma, dry mouth and skin, and cardiac arrhythmias.

Peppermint oil derivatives are associated with fewer unwanted effects, which are principally limited to symptoms of upper gastrointestinal disturbances. These have been reduced with the introduction of delayed release capsules.

Mebeverine hydrochloride and alverine citrate, like peppermint oil, are thought to achieve their antispasmodic effects by a direct relaxant action on intestinal smooth muscle. Their therapeutic benefit is uncertain, although unwanted side effects are less common than with anti-muscarinic and peppermint oil preparations.

Anti-inflammatory and immunomodulating drugs

Anti-inflammatory drugs are of principal value in inflammatory bowel diseases. Immunomodulating agents may also have a role in colitis and in colorectal cancer.

Steroid preparations

Steroids may be taken orally, rectally, parenterally, or topically. Oral steroids may be of value in active disease of moderate severity. Prednisolone is the most widely used preparation and the enteric coated formulation is commonly used, although there is little evidence that this reduces the adverse effects. Initial dosage may be high (for example, 30–60 mg/day), but courses of steroids should be kept as short as possible and the dose gradually reduced at the earliest opportunity.

Systemic side effects remain the major complication of steroid therapy in inflammatory bowel disease. Budesonide, a steroid preparation used widely in the treatment of asthma and rhinitis, has been recently adapted for use in ileocolonic Crohn's disease. When taken orally in a controlled release formulation, the drug acts topically in the ileum and right colon but, in contrast to prednisolone, over 90% of the drug is removed from the liver on first pass. Although budesonide has been shown to be effective as prednisolone in inducing symptomatic remission in ileocolonic Crohn's disease, the incidence of steroid induced side effects is significantly reduced. Budesonide treatment (which is limited to an eight week period) is significantly more expensive than prednisolone.

There is no evidence that continuous, low dose steroids reduce the risk of relapse in ulcerative colitis. Intravenous or intramuscular corticosteroids should be restricted to those cases of severe colitis that have failed to settle with oral steroids. In some cases high doses of steroids (100 mg hydrocortisone four times a day) may be of benefit, but patients should be monitored extremely closely for signs of acute toxic dilatation and converted to oral preparations as soon as their condition permits.

In contrast with systemic therapy, topical local steroid treatment may control proctitis or distal colitis, with a much reduced risk of the effects associated with systemic absorption, although a degree of systemic absorption does occur. Liquid (Predsol) and foam (Predfoam, Colifoam) enemas are available, in metered dose formulations. The foam is easy to retain and therefore suitable for daytime use. Steroid liquid enemas are more likely to be acceptable for nocturnal use and may reach more proximally within the colon. Steroid suppositories are less widely used than enemas but may be valuable in proctitis.

Some topical steroids are formulated as metasulphobenzoate salts to reduce their systemic absorption.

5-Aminosalicylic acid derivatives

There are several examples of drugs that contain 5-aminosalicylic acid, which reduces inflammation by a direct effect on colonic mucosa. In each case the active moiety is the acid, but the formulations differ in the way that the acid is delivered to the colon. The active moiety is associated with several adverse effects, including diarrhoea, nephritis, and salicylate hypersensitivity.

Sulphasalazine uses a carrier compound, sulphapyridine, to prevent absorption in the upper gastrointestinal tract. After metabolism by colonic bacteria 5-aminosalicylic acid is released within the colon. The carrier is associated with a high risk of adverse symptoms, including rashes, nausea and vomiting, blood dyscrasia, and azoospermia. Newer preparations such as olsalazine and mesalazine avoid this problem by altering the mechanism of delivery. In the case of olsalazine, two molecules of 5-aminosalicylic acid are coupled and the bond between them is cleaved in the colon. Asacol, a mesalazine preparation, uses a coat carrier which releases the 5-aminosalicylic acid when the pH of the gut lumen approaches 7. Pentasa, another mesalazine tablet, disintegrates in the stomach, releasing coated slow release granules. The granules then start releasing 5-aminosalicylic acid. Mesalazine preparations seem more promising in ileal Crohn's disease and right sided colitis, whereas osalazine may be more effective in left sided colitis.

Topical 5-aminosalicylic acid preparations such as mesalazine enemas are less likely to cause adverse effects, and may be used as an alternative to topical steroids. They are useful in distal colitis refractory to steroids.

5-Aminosalicylic acid preparations are moderately beneficial both to active disease and to maintain remission in ulcerative colitis. There is less evidence that they are of value in Crohn's disease.

Immunomodulating agents

Azathioprine—Azathioprine is rapidly and extensively metabolised to 6-mercaptopurine. Both drugs are available but azathioprine, because of its more predictable absorption, is the drug of choice. Patients should be informed that treatment takes up to 6–12 weeks to work. Azathioprine may allow the dose of steroids to be reduced in patients with long term disease who have frequent symptomatic relapses. Patients in whom steroids have unacceptable adverse effects should also be considered for this treatment.

The use of azathioprine should be restricted to specialist units in view of its considerable toxicity. The most common side effect is myelosuppression, though hepatic and pancreatic toxicity is also well recognised. Treatment should be started gradually with frequent (weekly) full blood counts during the first month. The frequency of monitoring can then be reduced to four to six times weekly for as long as the patient takes the drug.

Cyclosporin A—This has been evaluated in Crohn's disease. There is a variable response rate and its use should be guided by the considerations outlined for azathioprine. Unlike other immunosuppressive drugs it has little effect on bone marrow, its major adverse effect being nephrotoxicity. Renal function and plasma cyclosporin levels must be monitored closely during treatment.

Levamisole—A small but well controlled study has shown no benefit over placebo in Crohn's disease. There is evidence to suggest that when combined with fluorouracil as adjuvant

therapy for colorectal cancer significant improvements in five year survival occur in patients with lymph node metastases.

Cytotoxic drugs

The role of cytotoxic chemotherapy in metastatic colorectal cancer is unclear and results of studies to date have been disappointing. There is good evidence, however, of a survival advantage for patients with Dukes' C carcinoma given adjuvant postoperative chemotherapy with 5-fluorouracil and levamisole or folinic acid. The place of adjuvant chemotherapy in Dukes' B carcinoma is less clear and the QUASAR trial aims to answer this question.

Chemotherapy has transformed the treatment of anal cancer and made abdominoperineal resection unnecessary in most cases. A combination of mitomycin C, 5-fluorouracil, and radiotherapy allows 75% of patients with squamous carcinoma of the anus to be treated effectively without a colostomy.

In all cases, patients should be monitored carefully for mucositis and bone marrow suppression.

Antimicrobial drugs

There is a limited place for antimicrobial drugs in colorectal disease. Acute infective diarrhoea is, in general, not an indication for antibiotics, which may cause diarrhoea themselves. Important exceptions to this are the management of salmonella or campylobacter infection in elderly people and young children. For salmonellosis, ciprofloxacin is the drug of choice in adults, but in children and adults with a history of epilepsy a third generation cephalosporin should be used.

Pseudomembranous colitis, which commonly complicates the use of broad spectrum antibiotics, should always be considered in patients with diarrhoea after or during antibiotic treatment and in patients in intensive care units. It can occasionally be implicated in relapses in patients with inflammatory bowel disease. Oral metronidazole or vancomycin is effective in the management. Careful monitoring of these patients is required because severe cases may progress to acute toxic dilatation of the colon. In patients with fulminant colitis, significant amounts of vancomycin may be absorbed owing to alterations in the mucosal permeability of the inflamed colon, thus putting the patient at risk of ototoxicity and nephrotoxicity.

Protozoal and helminthic infection are clear indications for chemotherapy. Intestinal amoebiasis will respond to metronidazole or tinidazole and initial treatment should be followed by a 10 day course of diloxanide furoate, which will eliminate the cyst forms and render the patient less likely to develop chronic amoebiasis and to infect others.

Unlike intestinal amoebiasis, worm infestation is common in the United Kingdom. Threadworms and roundworms may infest whole households but respond to piperazine and mebendazole respectively. Reinfection is common, however, and patients may require several courses of therapy over a number of weeks, with careful and repeated examination of the stools.

As outlined above, the place of antimicrobial drugs is less well established. Inflammatory conditions such as Crohn's disease and ulcerative colitis do not require antimicrobial drugs. Metronidazole may be of value in perineal Crohn's disease, where local suppuration may be a problem. It has a role in patients with relapses of Crohn's colitis but is not suitable for long term use because of the likelihood of developing peripheral neuropathy.

Antibiotic prophylaxis for colorectal surgery

The current *British National Formulary*'s recommendation for antibiotic prophylaxis for colorectal surgery is a single dose of gentamicin and metronidazole, or cefuroxime and metronidazole given two hours before the operation. Both of these regimens will ensure therapeutic tissue concentrations against the common colorectal organisms at the start of the operation. As a result of practical considerations prophylaxis is often given at induction, which appears to be satisfactory. Antibiotics given after the initial incision must be considered to provide unsatisfactory prophylactic cover. A single dose is effective and further doses are indicated only if considerable faecal contamination occurs.

As a single dose is being given, reducing the dose of gentamicin to avoid renal impairment is unnecessary, and concerns about renal toxicity and ototoxicity unfounded.

Topical therapy

Three class of drugs are widely prescribed for haemorrhoids, pruritus ani, and anal fissure. All are of uncertain efficacy.

- Soothing creams such as anusol, which contains bismuth subgallate, a mild astringent
- Steroid preparations
- Local anaesthetic preparations.

These preparations are best avoided as there is little evidence of any benefit. They may cause maceration of the anal skin and aggravate pruritus ani.

Index

Index

Index

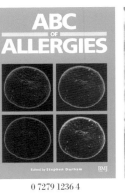
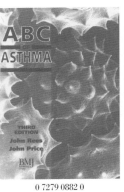
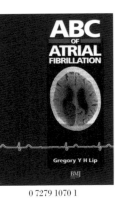

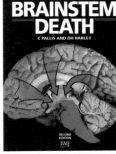
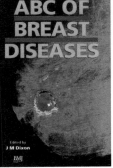
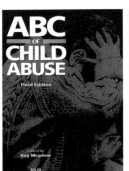
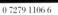
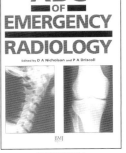
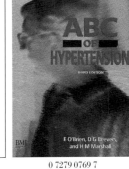
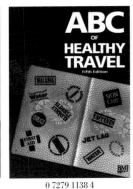
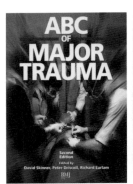
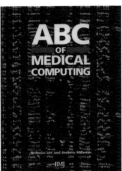
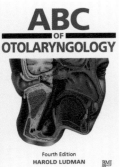
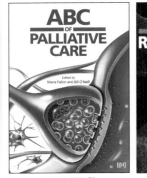
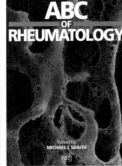
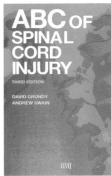
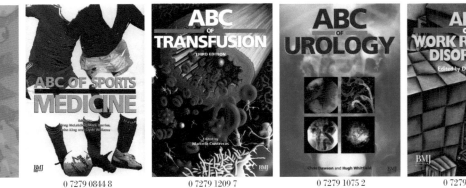
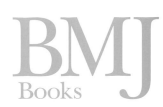